T0229003

Congenital and Acquired Disorders of Macrophages and Histiocytes

Editors

NANCY BERLINER
BARRETT J. ROLLINS

HEMATOLOGY/ONCOLOGY CLINICS OF NORTH AMERICA

www.hemonc.theclinics.com

Consulting Editors
GEORGE P. CANELLOS
H. FRANKLIN BUNN

October 2015 • Volume 29 • Number 5

ELSEVIER

1600 John F. Kennedy Boulevard • Suite 1800 • Philadelphia, Pennsylvania, 19103-2899

http://www.theclinics.com

HEMATOLOGY/ONCOLOGY CLINICS OF NORTH AMERICA Volume 29, Number 5
October 2015 ISSN 0889-8588, ISBN 13: 978-0-323-40088-6

Editor: Jennifer Flynn-Briggs
Developmental Editor: Kristen Helm

Hematology/Oncology Clinics (ISSN 0889-8588) is published bimonthly by Elsevier Inc., 360 Park Avenue South, New York, NY 10010-1710. Months of issue are February, April, June, August, October, and December. Business and Editorial Offices: 1600 John F. Kennedy Blvd., Ste. 1800, Philadelphia, PA 19103–2899. Customer Service Office: 3251 Riverport Lane, Maryland Heights, MO 63043. Periodicals postage paid at New York, NY and at additional mailing offices. Subscription prices are $385.00 per year (domestic individuals), $633.00 per year (domestic institutions), $190.00 per year (domestic students/residents), $440.00 per year (Canadian individuals), $783.00 per year (Canadian institutions) $520.00 per year (international individuals), $783.00 per year (international institutions), and $255.00 per year (international and Canadian students/residents). International air speed delivery is included in all *Clinics* subscription prices. All prices are subject to change without notice. **POSTMASTER:** Send address changes to *Hematology/Oncology Clinics of North America*, Elsevier Health Sciences Division, Subscription Customer Service, 3251 Riverport Lane, Maryland Heights, MO 63043. Customer Service (orders, claims, online, change of address): Elsevier Health Sciences Division, Subscription **Customer Service, 3251 Riverport Lane, Maryland Heights, MO 63043. Tel: 1-800-654-2452 (U.S. and Canada); 314-447-8871 (outside U.S. and Canada). Fax: 314-447-8029. E-mail: journalscustomerservice-usa@elsevier.com (for print support); journalsonlinesupport-usa@elsevier.com (for online support).**

Reprints. For copies of 100 or more, of articles in this publication, please contact the Commercial Reprints Department, Elsevier Inc., 360 Park Avenue South, New York, New York 10010-1710; Tel.: 212-633-3874, Fax: 212-633-3820, E-mail: reprints@elsevier.com.

Hematology/Oncology Clinics of North America is covered in *MEDLINE/PubMed (Index Medicus), EMBASE/ Excerpta Medica,* and *BIOSIS.*

Contributors

CONSULTING EDITORS

GEORGE P. CANELLOS, MD
William Rosenberg Professor of Medicine, Department of Medical Oncology, Dana-Farber Cancer Institute, Boston, Massachusetts

H. FRANKLIN BUNN, MD
Professor of Medicine, Division of Hematology, Brigham and Women's Hospital, Harvard Medical School, Boston, Massachusetts

EDITORS

NANCY BERLINER, MD
Chief, Division of Hematology, Brigham and Women's Hospital; Professor of Medicine, Harvard Medical School, Boston, Massachusetts

BARRETT J. ROLLINS, MD, PhD
Chief Scientific Officer, Department of Medical Oncology, Dana-Farber Cancer Institute; Linde Family Professor of Medicine, Department of Medicine, Brigham and Women's Hospital, Harvard Medical School, Boston, Massachusetts

AUTHORS

CARL E. ALLEN, MD, PhD
Texas Children's Cancer Center, Baylor College of Medicine, Houston, Texas

†ROBERT J. ARCECI, MD, PhD
Director, Children's Center for Cancer and Blood Disorders; Director of the Ron Matricaria Institute of Molecular Medicine, Department of Child Health, Phoenix Children's Hospital, University of Arizona College of Medicine, Phoenix, Arizona

NANCY BERLINER, MD
Chief, Division of Hematology, Brigham and Women's Hospital; Professor of Medicine, Harvard Medical School, Boston, Massachusetts

VENETIA BIGLEY, MD, PhD
Human Dendritic Cell Laboratory, Institute of Cellular Medicine, Newcastle University, Newcastle upon Tyne, United Kingdom

MEGHAN CAMPO, MD
Clinical Hematology Oncology Fellow, Dana-Farber Cancer Institue, Boston, Massachusetts

---

†Deceased.

SHANMUGANATHAN CHANDRAKASAN, MD
Immunodeficiency and Histiocytosis Program, Cancer and Blood Diseases Institute, Cincinnati Children's Hospital Medical Center, Cincinnati, Ohio

MATTHEW COLLIN, MD, PhD
Human Dendritic Cell Laboratory, Institute of Cellular Medicine, Newcastle University, Newcastle upon Tyne, United Kingdom

RANDY Q. CRON, MD, PhD
Professor of Pediatrics and Medicine, Arthritis Foundation, Alabama Chapter; Endowed Chair; Director, Division of Pediatric Rheumatology, Children's Hospital of Alabama and University of Alabama at Birmingham, Birmingham, Alabama

SERGIO DAVÌ, MD
Research Fellow, Second Pediatric Division and Rheumatology, G. Gaslini Institute, Genoa, Italy

BARBARA DEGAR, MD
Assistant Professor, Harvard Medical School; Senior Physician, Pediatric Oncology, Dana-Farber/Boston Children's Cancer and Blood Disorders Center, Boston, Massachusetts

ALEXANDRA H. FILIPOVICH, MD
Immunodeficiency and Histiocytosis Program, Cancer and Blood Diseases Institute, Cincinnati Children's Hospital Medical Center, Cincinnati, Ohio

SHINSAKU IMASHUKU, MD, PhD
Consultant of Hematology and Pediatrics, Division of Hematology, Takasago-Seibu Hospital, Takasago, Japan

RONALD JAFFE, MB, BCh
Department of Pathology, Magee-Womens Hospital of UPMC, University of Pittsburgh School of Medicine, Pittsburgh, Pennsylvania

ALBERTO MARTINI, MD
Professor of Pediatrics; Head, Department of Pediatrics and Second Pediatric Division and Rheumatology, University of Genoa and G. Gaslini Institute; Chairman of the Pediatric Rheumatology European Society (PRES) and the Pediatric Rheumatology International Trials Organization (PRINTO), Genoa, Italy

KENNETH L. McCLAIN, MD, PhD
Texas Children's Cancer Center, Baylor College of Medicine, Houston, Texas

FRANCESCA MINOIA, MD
Medical Assistant, Second Pediatric Division and Rheumatology, G. Gaslini Institute, Genoa, Italy

CHALINEE MONSEREENUSORN, MD
Department of Pediatric Oncology, Dana-Farber/Boston Children's Cancer and Blood Disorders Center, Boston, Massachusetts

SARAH NIKIFOROW, MD, PhD
Clinical Instructor, Stem Cell Transplantation Program, Cell Manipulation Core Facility, Dana-Farber Cancer Institute, Boston, Massachusetts

JENNIFER PICARSIC, MD
Department of Pathology, Children's Hospital of Pittsburgh of UPMC, University of Pittsburgh School of Medicine, Pittsburgh, Pennsylvania

ANGELO RAVELLI, MD
Associate Professor of Pediatrics, Department of Neuroscience, Rehabilitation, Ophthalmology, Genetics, Maternal and Child Health; Head, Center of Rheumatology, University of Genoa and G. Gaslini Institute, Genoa, Italy

CARLOS RODRIGUEZ-GALINDO, MD
Department of Pediatric Oncology, Dana-Farber/Boston Children's Cancer and Blood Disorders Center; Department of Pediatrics, Harvard Medical School, Boston, Massachusetts

BARRETT J. ROLLINS, MD, PhD
Chief Scientific Officer, Department of Medical Oncology, Dana-Farber Cancer Institute; Linde Family Professor of Medicine, Department of Medicine, Brigham and Women's Hospital, Harvard Medical School, Boston, Massachusetts

Contents

The classification of the histiocytoses has evolved based on new understanding of the cell of origin as a bone marrow precursor. Although the pathologic features of the histiocytoses have not changed per se, molecular genetic information now needs to be integrated into the diagnosis. The basic lesions of the most common histiocytoses, their patterns in different sites, and ancillary diagnostics are now just one part of the classification. As more is understood about the cell of origin and molecular biology of the histiocytoses, future classifications will be refined.

Langerhans cell histiocytosis (LCH) is a heterogeneous disease characterized by common histology of inflammatory lesions containing Langerin+ (CD207) histiocytes. Emerging data support a model in which MAPK activation in self-renewing hematopoietic progenitors may drive disseminated high-risk disease, whereas MAPK activation in more differentiated committed myeloid populations may induce low-risk LCH. The heterogeneous clinical manifestations with shared histology may represent the final common pathway of an acquired defect of differentiation, initiated at more than one point. Implications of this model include re-definition of LCH as a myeloid neoplasia and re-focusing therapeutic strategies on the cells and lineages of origin.

The discovery of recurrent somatic genomic alterations in Langerhans cell histiocytosis (LCH) has led to a new understanding of LCH as a clonal neoplastic disorder. Most of the abnormalities described to date affect the RAS/RAF/MEK/extracellular-signal-regulated kinase (ERK) pathway: more than 50% of LCH cases carry activating mutations in *BRAF*, whereas another 10% to 28% carry activating mutations of *MAP2K1*, which encodes MEK1. The pathogenetic importance of these mutations has been confirmed by reports of significant clinical responses to RAF inhibitors.

Langerhans cell histiocytosis (LCH) is a disease caused by clonal prolifer-ation of CD1a+/CD207+ cells that is characterized by a spectrum of vary-ing degrees of organ involvement and dysfunction. Treatment of LCH is risk adapted; patients with single lesions may respond well to local treat-ment, whereas patients with multi-system disease and risk-organ involve-ment require more intensive therapy. Although survival for patients without organ dysfunction is excellent, mortality rates for patients with organ dysfunction may reach 30% to 40%. For patients with low-risk disease, although cure is almost universal, disease reactivation rates are in excess of 30%.

Diseases of the central nervous system (CNS) are common in patients with Langerhans cell histiocytosis (LCH). Besides active LCH lesions, neurode-generative (ND) lesions of the cerebellum and/or basal ganglia may occur as late sequelae of LCH. While the etiology of this ND disease remains un-clear, biomarkers in cerebrospinal fluid (CSF) may reflect the activity of CNS disease in these patients. However, no well-planned CSF studies have yet been performed in patients at high risk for ND-CNS-LCH. Poten-tial parallels with other neuroinflammatory/neurodegenerative diseases suggest the utility of examining these other disorders in establishing stra-tegies for the prevention and/or treatment of ND-CNS-LCH.

Hemophagocytic Lymphohistiocytosis (HLH), an inherited life-threatening inflammatory disorder, has gained growing recognition not only in children but also increasingly in adults over the past 2 decades. HLH involves inborn defects in lymphocytes, which normally mediate control of infec-tious and inflammatory conditions within the immune system and in other tissues. In the context of inherited defects in cytotoxic cells and other im-mune cells, the disorder is classified as familial or primary HLH. Secondary HLH occurs in the settings of infections or underlying rheumatologic disor-ders. Secondary HLH also accompanies some lymphoid malignancies.

Familial hemophagocytic lymphohistiocytosis (FHL) is a rare heritable dis-order of immune regulation that is typically characterized by sudden onset of severe systemic illness. Functional impairment or absence of 1 or more of several proteins that participate in lymphocyte cytotoxicity underlies the disease. Although FHL usually presents in infancy, age of onset is variable and dependent on genetic and environmental factors. Initial treatment consists of immune suppression, whereas definitive treatment requires hematopoietic cell transplantation.

Hemophagocytic lymphohistiocytosis (HLH) is a rare but potentially fatal syndrome of pathologic immune dysregulation characterized by clinical signs and symptoms of extreme inflammation. HLH can occur as a genetic or sporadic disorder and, though seen as an inherited condition affecting primarily a pediatric population, can occur at any age and can be encountered in association with a variety of underlying diseases. Clinically, the syndrome, whether genetic or acquired, is characterized by fever, hepatosplenomegaly, cytopenias, and activated macrophages in hematopoietic organs. Therapy centers on suppression of this hyperinflammatory state with cytotoxic, immunosuppressive therapy and treatment of any existing HLH triggers.

Macrophage activation syndrome (MAS) is a potentially life-threatening complication of rheumatic disorders that occurs most commonly in systemic juvenile idiopathic arthritis. In recent years, there have been several advances in the understanding of the pathophysiology of MAS. Furthermore, new classification criteria have been developed. Although the place of cytokine blockers in the management of MAS is still unclear, interleukin-1 inhibitors represent a promising adjunctive therapy, particularly in refractory cases.

The role of reduced-intensity allogeneic hematopoietic stem cell transplantation (HSCT) from a variety of donor sources in improving survival for children with familial hemophagocytic lymphohistiocytosis (HLH) is well-documented. The heterogeneity of adult-onset HLH has complicated evaluation of initial therapy and of HSCT as definitive treatment. Therapy for adults with HLH is often individualized, but institutions are now generating algorithms that include HSCT based on growing experience. Consolidation of these data is needed to optimize management of the growing number of adults recognized to have HLH and to achieve dramatic improvements in survival.

HEMATOLOGY/ONCOLOGY
CLINICS OF NORTH AMERICA

Dedication

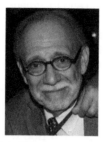

Robert J. Arceci, MD, PhD at a recent Nikolas Symposium

This issue of the *Hematology/Oncology Clinics of North America* is dedicated to the memory of Dr Bob Arceci, who died tragically in a motorcycle accident only one day after submitting his contribution to this series. Bob was one of the world's leading pediatric oncologists and was not only a compassionate clinician but also a dedicated clinical and translational researcher of the leukemias and myeloid neoplasms of childhood.

Bob received his MD and PhD from the University of Rochester and completed his residency in pediatrics at Boston Children's Hospital. He was then a fellow in pediatric hematology and oncology in the combined program at Boston Children's and Dana-Farber Cancer Institute, where many of us first came to know him. There followed a series of major leadership roles in pediatrics and pediatric hematology/oncology, including division chief at Cincinnati Children's Hospital Medical Center, then King Fahd Professor of Pediatric Oncology, and director of the division at Johns Hopkins School of Medicine. In 2013, he moved to the University of Arizona, where he was Professor of Pediatrics, Director of the Children's Center for Cancer and Blood Disorders, and Co-Director of the Ron Matricaria Institute of Molecular Medicine at Phoenix Children's Hospital. The latter position was very important to Bob, who had become increasingly interested in using the molecular abnormalities of malignant disease to guide precision therapy. Bob was also committed to the pediatric oncology community and provided guidance and leadership to entities such as the Children's Oncology Group, the Children's Cancer Group, the Pediatric Oncology Group, and the St. Baldrick's Foundation, where he was on the Board of Directors and chair of the Scientific Advisory Committee.

At the time of his death, Bob was editor-in-chief of *Pediatric Blood and Cancer*. He had also served as editor-in-chief of the *Journal of Pediatric Hematology/Oncology* and associate editor of the *Journal of Pediatrics*. He was co-editor of several influential textbooks, including *Pediatric Hematology, Molecularly Targeted Therapy for Childhood Cancer, Cancer Genomics: From Bench to Personalized Medicine*, and section editor for the neoplastic disorders portion of Rudolph's *Pediatrics*.

In addition to all of these accomplishments, Bob was a charismatic figure who could twist your arm in the name of a good cause and get you to work hard on one of his

Hematol Oncol Clin N Am 29 (2015) xi–xii
http://dx.doi.org/10.1016/j.hoc.2015.07.002
0889-8588/15/$ – see front matter © 2015 Published by Elsevier Inc.

hemonc.theclinics.com

xii   Dedication

projects all the while thinking it was your own idea to participate. Most famously and wonderfully, he helped direct the Nikolas Symposium, a yearly "think tank" held in Greece and devoted to advancing the understanding and treatment of the histiocytoses. Founded by Paul Kontoyannis and his family, the Symposia are named for Paul's son Nikolas, who had Langerhans cell histiocytosis as a child and now suffers from its sequelae. The Symposium, which recently held its 25th annual meeting, is designed to attract a small number of scientists and clinicians from widely diverse fields to talk about this challenging and enigmatic disease.

Getting prominent and busy people to commit to meeting in Athens for a week about a rare disease is a daunting task, but Bob was exactly the right person for the job. His buoyant enthusiasm, infectious laugh, and undiminished curiosity motivated everyone to participate at their highest level. It also didn't hurt that Bob was an unabashed dancer and a vigorous if not always tonally precise singer. He was instrumental in turning the social events at the Nikolas Symposia into memorable and, frankly, legendary nights.

Bob also had enthusiasms that he loved to share. One was for opera. Another was for motorcycles, about which he famously said that all other vehicles are "just transportation." We will miss Bob terribly. The world is a better place for his having been part of it, and we are better people for having known him.

Barrett J. Rollins, MD, PhD

Carl E. Allen, MD

Matthew Collin, MD, PhD

Ronald Jaffe, MD, BCh

Jennifer L. Picarsic, MD

Carlos Rodriguez-Galindo, MD

E-mail address:
barrett_rollins@dfci.harvard.edu (B.J. Rollins)

Preface

Congenital and Acquired Disorders of Macrophages and Histiocytes

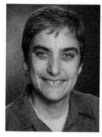 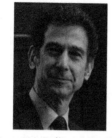

Nancy Berliner, MD   Barrett J. Rollins, MD, PhD
Editors

Histiocytes are bone marrow–derived cells that protect the body from foreign substances by phagocytosing them and, in some cases, using the engulfed material to stimulate an immune response. Unlike circulating monocytes, histiocytes are found in tissues, although some can migrate to lymph nodes and other sites following stimulation. The histiocytoses, then, are diseases that are characterized by the uncontrolled accumulation of histiocytes with attendant tissue damage. Broadly, they can be divided into three categories based on their cell of origin and their behavior: (1) those whose abnormal cells resemble dendritic cells, including Langerhans cell histiocytosis (LCH), Erdheim-Chester disease, and juvenile xanthogranuloma; (2) those whose abnormal cells resemble macrophages, including hemophagocytic lymphohistiocytosis (HLH) and Rosai-Dorfman disease; and (3) malignant histiocytoses. This issue of the *Hematology/Oncology Clinics of North America* presents new information on diseases in the first two categories.

The very first issue of this series, from 1987, reviewed the state of knowledge about what was then called Histiocytosis X. At that time, the most important advances involved the understanding that a single cell type, one which resembled a mature Langerhans cell, was present in the myriad forms of the disease. Although the disease could now be called LCH, its fundamental nature remained a puzzle. Eleven years later, another issue in this series, edited by Maarten Egeler and Giulio D'Angio, provided an update that was remarkable for integrating the new finding that the cells in LCH are clonal, suggesting that LCH might be a neoplasm. However, a mechanistic understanding of its pathogenesis was still unavailable. The current issue is focused on a series of recent advances that begin to reveal the true nature of LCH and provide some therapeutic targets. In particular:

Hematol Oncol Clin N Am 29 (2015) xiii–xv
http://dx.doi.org/10.1016/j.hoc.2015.07.001
0889-8588/15/$ – see front matter © 2015 Published by Elsevier Inc.

hemonc.theclinics.com

1. Recurrent genomic abnormalities. Dr Rollins and Drs Picarsic and Jaffe discuss the new understanding of LCH as a neoplastic disease based on the presence of somatic mutations in components of the RAS-RAF-MEK-ERK pathway in the majority of patients. Drs Monsereenusorn and Rodriguez-Galindo discuss current treatment as well as the implications of these actionable mutations in the future treatment of LCH.
2. Cell of origin. Drs Collin, Bigley, McClain, and Allen discuss recent findings indicating that LCH is most likely a neoplasm of myeloid progenitors rather than Langerhans cells and the implications this has for treatment and diagnosis.
3. Clinical treatment. Drs Monsereenusorn and Rodriguez-Galindo present an up-to-date summary of the standard and experimental approaches to LCH treatment, and our late colleague, Dr Bob Arceci, and his coauthor, Dr Imashuku, describe the state of knowledge about neurodegeneration in LCH, a devastating concomitant in many cases.

The previously mentioned 1998 issue of *Hematology/Oncology Clinics of North America* included articles on the relatively newly described entity of HLH. At that time, HLH was a clinical syndrome that had been identified as a primary hereditary disease in infants and young children, and as an acquired disease associated with infection, autoimmune disease, and malignancy. At that time, the pathophysiologic basis for the disease was unknown. The intervening years have witnessed an explosion of information about the natural history of the disease and its molecular underpinnings. In this issue of the *Hematology/Oncology Clinics of North America*, we include a series of reviews summarizing the state of our knowledge of HLH. These reflect the growing awareness of the unexpectedly common occurrence of this disorder in older age groups, as well as our current understanding of the molecular basis for familial HLH and its relationship to the acquired forms seen in patients of all ages:

1. Pathogenesis of HLH. Drs Filipovich and Chandrakasan discuss the pathophysiology of HLH with regard to the immune pathways that are dysregulated in the disease. They discuss the identified molecular lesions that underlie the familial form of the disease, and also the increasing understanding of the role of molecular defects in acquired forms of HLH.
2. Familial HLH. Dr Degar discusses the pathophysiologic and clinical features of HLH as seen in young children. She presents the current approach to diagnosis and treatment of the disease as seen in the pediatric age group.
3. HLH in adults. Drs Campo and Berliner present the features of the increasingly recognized syndrome of HLH as seen in adult patients, emphasizing the role of hypomorphic alleles of familial HLH genes in its pathogenesis, the frequent association with lymphoproliferative malignancy, and the necessity of early intervention in this otherwise rapidly fatal syndrome.
4. Macrophage activation syndrome. Drs Ravelli, Davì, Minoia, Martini, and Cron discuss the features of HLH as seen in association with systemic autoimmune diseases, especially systemic lupus erythematosis and juvenile inflammatory arthritis. They emphasize the distinctly different natural history, prognosis, and treatment approaches to this variant of HLH in comparison to the other acquired forms of the disease.
5. Stem cell transplant for HLH. Stem cell transplant is the only curative approach to familial HLH and may represent the best option for many patients with the acquired form of the disease as well. Dr Nikiforow details the clinical approach to

transplantation across the spectrum of HLH patients, including considerations of donor choice, preparative regimens, and timing of transplant to optimize outcomes.

Nancy Berliner, MD
Division of Hematology
Brigham and Women's Hospital
Harvard Medical School
Mid-Campus 3
75 Francis Street
Boston, MA 02115, USA

Barrett J. Rollins, MD, PhD
Department of Medical Oncology
Dana-Farber Cancer Institute
Department of Medicine
Brigham & Women's Hospital
Harvard Medical School
450 Brookline Avenue
Boston, MA 02215, USA

E-mail addresses:
nberliner@partners.org (N. Berliner)
barrett_rollins@dfci.harvard.edu (B.J. Rollins)

Nosology and Pathology of Langerhans Cell Histiocytosis

Jennifer Picarsic, MD[a],*, Ronald Jaffe, MB, BCh[b]

KEYWORDS

- Langerhans cell histocytosis • Juvenile xanthogranuloma • Rosai-Dorfman disease
- Erdheim-Chester disease • Congenital and acquired disorders

KEY POINTS

- The histopathology and immunophenotype of the histiocytoses define the various families of lesions, LCH, JXG, ECD, and RDD.
- LCH is defined by histopathology and the immunophenotype CD1a/CD207 (Langerin)/S100 and the BRAF V600E mutation in more than half of cases.
- JXG is defined by histopathology and the immunophenotype CD14/CD68/CD163/Factor 13a/fascin but little S100 and no CD1a/CD207 or *BRAF* mutations.
- ECD is defined by clinical/radiographic features and JXG-type pathology with the BRAF V600E mutation in more than half of cases.
- RDD is defined by its histopathology with the RDD cell being selectively S100/fascin-positive.
- Understanding the cell of origin and integration of the molecular biology helps to further define these histiocytic lesions going forward, especially in cases where diagnostic LCH cells are not found.

PATHOLOGY OF THE HISTIOCYTOSES

Current practice is to categorize the histiocytoses based on their histopathology into three basic families: (1) Langerhans cell histiocytosis (LCH), (2) juvenile xanthogranuloma family (JXG), and (3) Rosai-Dorfman disease (RDD). The histopathology superimposed with the clinical features and staging of the condition results in a final diagnosis, which accounts for most histiocytosis. There are instances of combined lesions either

The authors have no commercial or financial conflicts of interest to disclose.
[a] Department of Pathology, Children's Hospital of Pittsburgh of UPMC, University of Pittsburgh School of Medicine, One Children's Hospital Drive, 4401 Penn Avenue, Pittsburgh, PA 15224, USA; [b] Department of Pathology, Magee-Womens Hospital of UPMC, University of Pittsburgh School of Medicine, 300 Halket St., Pittsburgh, PA 15213, USA
* Corresponding author. Department of Pathology, Children's Hospital of Pittsburgh of UPMC, One Children's Hospital Drive, 4401 Penn Avenue, Main Hospital, B260, Pittsburgh, PA 15224.
E-mail address: picarsicj@upmc.edu

Hematol Oncol Clin N Am 29 (2015) 799–823
http://dx.doi.org/10.1016/j.hoc.2015.06.001
0889-8588/15/$ – see front matter © 2015 Elsevier Inc. All rights reserved.

within the same site or at different sites in the same patient, which suggest that the histopathologic distinction does not strictly conform to the biology. This is best seen with LCH and Erdheim-Chester disease (ECD), which shares the histopathology of the JXG family; both conditions can occur in the same patient and both have a high incidence of *BRAF* mutations, even though these mutations are not a feature of the JXG family as a whole.[1] Combined LCH and RDD or LCH and JXG in the same patient are increasingly recognized.[2–4] Other more unusual histiocytic lesions include the LCH-like indeterminate cell histiocytosis, characterized by the presence of CD1a but a lack of CD207 or Birbeck granules.[5] There are an insufficient number of cases to draw broad biologic conclusions that they differ markedly from LCH. A JXG-like systemic histiocytosis is the ALK-positive histiocytosis, most commonly in young females. It is defined by the presence of *ALK* mutations, including a rare example with a *TPM3-ALK* transcript.[6] Again, there are too few cases for broad generalizations. For the purposes of this article, the pathology of the main histiocytoses families is contrasted, knowing that there is overlap.

GENERAL HISTOPATHOLOGY

Diagnosis of LCH requires a clonal neoplastic proliferation that expresses the immunohistochemical panel of CD1a, CD207 (Langerin), and S100 (**Fig. 1**). About 60% of cases have a BRAF V600E mutation.[7,8] The cells are generally large, 15 to 25 μm, round to

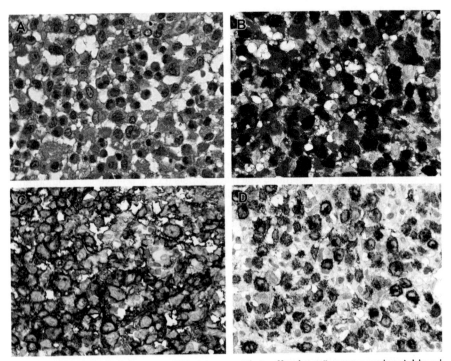

Fig. 1. (*A*) LCH cells with large oval histiocytes with "coffee-bean" groove and variable admixed eosinophils. (*B*) Nuclear and cytoplasmic S100 expression. (*C*) Surface and paranuclear CD1a expression. (*D*) Granular cytoplasmic CD207 (Langerin) expression. Hematoxylin and Eosin [H&E], original magnification ×1000.

oval in shape without the branching that characterizes inflammatory CD1a$^+$ dendritic cells. The nucleus has a complex contour with a "coffee-bean" nuclear groove (see **Fig. 1**). The CD207 immunostain has supplanted the need for electron microscopy (**Box 1**).[9,10] An inflammatory milieu of macrophages, eosinophils, and small lymphocytes is admixed with the LCH cells, but plasma cells are rare. Mitotic figures can at times be brisk but are not a cause for concern of Langerhans cell sarcoma unless there are atypical mitoses, marked pleomorphism, and frank cytologic atypia. LCH cells dual stained for Ki-67 and CD1a or CD207 have a proliferation rate of about 10% (Ronald Jaffe, MB,BCh, authors' personal observation, 1985–2015). The appearance of LCH can vary by site and age of the lesion. Diagnostic challenge ensues when LCH cells are replaced by a fibroxanthomatous/inflammatory picture (false negative) and in chronic inflammatory processes in which the presence of CD1a$^+$ dendritic cells can confound (false positive) (**Box 1**).

JXG has an oval nucleus, inconspicuous nucleolus, and a variable amount of eosinophilic cytoplasm. The cells are variably spindled with the presence of multinucleated Touton giant cells typically present. The early JXG cell is more epithelioid and becomes progressively lipidized. The reticulohistiocytoma (oncocytic) variant is a large cell with abundant deeply eosinophilic cytoplasm. A lymphocytic interspersed component and occasionally, eosinophils, is typical. The result is that the JXG family of lesions can have a variety of appearances. The immunophenotype is fairly consistent but may vary with time: CD14/CD68/CD163/Factor 13a/fascin are all strongly expressed, except in purely xanthomatous cells that retain only CD68. CD1a and CD207 are absent, with light and variable staining for S100 in about 20% of cases.[11] A panel is more convincing than any individual stain. The mitotic rate can vary, but is in the same range as LCH. A highly pleomorphic and cytologically atypical lesion with atypical mitoses but with the same immunophenotype is a histiocytic sarcoma with JXG phenotype.[12]

RDD may be a phenotype that is common to several clinical conditions. Nodal sinus histiocytosis with massive lymphadenopathy is the prototype but extranodal disease is seen in greater than 40% of cases. Areas of RDD-type pathology have been seen in patients with autoimmune lymphoproliferative syndrome, Hodgkin lymphoma, HIV, and LCH.[2,13–15] Plasma cells are usually abundant, and in about 20% of cases IgG4 predominance is found, with a possible association with IgG4-related disease in some cases.[16] The histopathology of the autoinflammatory condition caused by mutation of the nucleoside transporter SLC29A3 is also that of RDD.[17] The very large RDD cell has water-clear cytoplasm containing emperipolesis. Some RDD nuclei are very large, hypochromatic, and have a prominent nucleolus. The RDD cell selectively stains strongly for S100 and fascin in a cytoplasmic pattern that highlights the emperipolesis, with CD14/CD68 and variable CD163, whereas CD1a/CD207 are absent. Late RDD lesions are fibrosing and residual islands of RDD may be hard to find.[11] Unlike LCH and JXG, there is no malignant counterpart.

Box 1
Diagnostic features of LCH

- Large (15–25 μm) oval, nondendritic cellular proliferation
- Complex, folded nuclear contour with "coffee-bean" groove
- Surface/paranuclear CD1a, granular cytoplasmic CD207 (Langerin), nuclear, and cytoplasmic S100.

HISTOPATHOLOGY IN SPECIFIC ORGANS
Bone

Osseous involvement is the quintessential LCH lesion presenting as a single lytic lesion or as a multiostotic, single system (SS) disease, but may also present as part of multisystem (MS) disease. Lytic skull lesions, especially of the calvaria and temporal bones, are a favored site and often involve the adjacent dura. Other osseous involvement includes vertebrae, jaws, ribs, pelvic bones, and proximal longs bones, but small bones of the hands and feet are spared.[18] Involvement of central nervous system (CNS) "risk" bones (ie, temporal bones of the skull base, maxillofacial bones [sphenoid, ethmoid, and zygomatic], and orbital bones) are associated with higher risk of diabetes insipidus (DI), endocrinopathies, and/or CNS involvement, including late neurodegenerative sequelae.[18] Chronic otitis or mastoiditis may herald involvement of the temporal bone and proptosis is present with orbital lesions. Bone pain is a common presentation. Neurologic defects may be present with vertebral collapse/vertebra plana when there is compression of the spinal cord. Loose teeth should raise the possibility of jaw involvement.[18]

When undergoing biopsy procedures in the active phase, these lesions often show diffuse sheets of LCH cells and bone destruction (**Fig. 2**). Immunostains confirm the

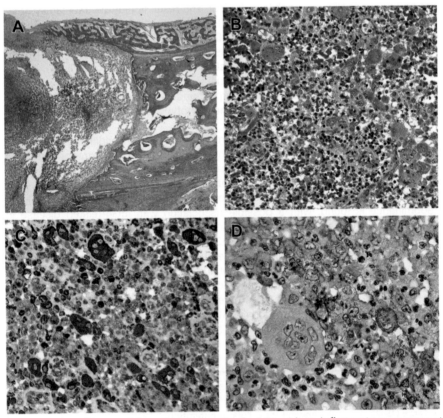

Fig. 2. (*A, B*) Skull bone with cortical destruction by LCH with an inflammatory component including osteoclast-like (OC) giant cells (*A*, Original magnification ×20; *B*, Original magnification ×400). (*C*) The OC-like giant cells are highlighted with CD68 (Original magnification ×400). (*D*) The LCH cells have occasional binucleation/multinucleation, highlighted by the CD1a immunostain, but the OC-like giant cells are negative (Original magnification ×1000).

diagnosis but rare cases may show only a minority of LCH cells displaying CD1a/CD207 (**Fig. 3**). Later lesions may involute with fibrosis, xanthomatous histiocytes, scattered inflammatory cells, and retain only small pockets of LCH cells. At times extensive fibrosis in the absence of LCH cells precludes a definite diagnosis and chronic osteomyelitis, fibrohistiocytic lesions, or JXG may be considered. An inflammatory milieu is admixed with LCH cells, with macrophages, eosinophils, and lymphocytes. Multinucleated osteoclastic giant cells may also be present, which lack the grooved nuclei of the binucleated/multinucleated LCH cell (see **Fig. 2**). Plasma cells are rare in active LCH, but may be present after a pathologic fracture making distinction from chronic osteomyelitis or chronic recurrent multifocal osteomyelitis impossible in the absence of LCH cells. Histologically LCH can occasionally undergo aneurysmal bone cyst change.[19]

RDD of the bone is usually diagnosed as an unexpected finding when LCH or osteomyelitis is suspected. It may cause initial confusion with LCH because of the S100+ cells but the large hypochromatic cells with emperipolesis should exclude LCH.

JXG can affect bones of any site and causes diagnostic confusion in the differential of a late sclerosing/involuting LCH lesion. It is usually part of a systemic JXG process and is rarely an isolated bone lesion. BRAF mutations are generally absent but the overlap with LCH is especially problematic in cases of JXG that develop after the treatment of LCH.[20] Berres and colleagues[8] showed two LCH cases in which subsequent pathology showed JXG pathology with a low level (0.03%–0.4%) of cells still showing a persistent BRAF V600E mutation. *BRAF* mutation status may provide better diagnostic clarity in the future for these challenging cases if the original LCH lesion was mutation positive.

ECD of bone is often suspected by virtue of the complicated clinical presentation with suggestive radiograph findings of bilateral long-bone osteosclerosis or retroperitoneal computed tomography/MRI findings. The histopathology of new lesions is that of a fibrosing lesion with the epithelioid JXG immunophenotype (CD14/CD68/CD163/F13a/fascin). CD1a and CD207 are absent, but S100 may be sparse and variable. Later lesions that are fibrotic and purely xanthomatous may have only CD68 expression. Like LCH, BRAF V600E mutation is seen in most cases.[21]

Skin

Skin rash is a common presentation of LCH. In children it presents as a persistent seborrheic dermatitis or papulonodular eruption involving flexures (axilla, groin, and so forth) and the scalp. In neonatal LCH, nodular skin lesions and rash are the most

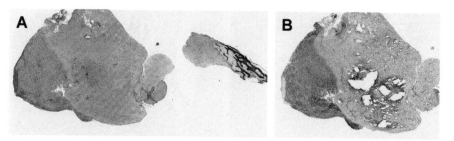

Fig. 3. Skull bone with nodule of LCH showing areas of necrosis, infiltrating through the bone into the soft tissue (*A*, H&E). This is an unusual case in that only a minority of cells stain for (*B*) CD1a (membranous) and CD207 (not shown). (Digital whole slide images (WSI) are hosted courtesy of University of Pittsburgh School of Medicine, Department of Pathology, Division of Informatics with permission.)

common presentation. Although some neonatal skin disease may spontaneously regress (so-called Hashimoto-Pritzker disease or self-healing reticulohistiocytosis), careful staging is necessary to know which cases may actually have MS involvement because the histopathology is not predictive.[22–24] Skin disease in adults is rare but presents as papulonodular eruptions or plaques over flexure sites and the scalp or as genital/perianal erosions.[25,26] In children and adults, SS involvement of the skin may be the only presentation, but careful staging is needed to rule out MS involvement.[25] In adults, skin LCH is also reported to have an increased risk of a subsequent hematologic malignancy.[26]

Diffuse sheets of LCH cells often fill the papillary and/or deeper dermis. Immunostains highlight the lesional cells especially in cases with overlying ulceration (**Fig. 4**). The differential diagnosis includes a chronic dermatitis with perivascular inflammation with a high content of CD1a$^+$/CD207$^-$ spindly dermal dendritic cells (**Fig. 5**), a consequence of chronic scabies and postinfectious conditions. Immune defects, such as Omenn syndrome (OMIM #603554), may have S100$^+$ dendritic cell hyperplasia. Nodular lesions should be distinguished from mastocytosis that expresses CD117 and tryptase. Immature myelomonocytic dermal infiltrates that express CD1a$^+$ are best diagnosed with a panel including CD14/lysozyme/MPO/CD68-KP1 (an early myeloid marker), and Ki-67, which is generally high.[27]

JXG of the skin is more common than LCH, presenting as dermal and sometimes deep nodules. The diagnosis is confirmed by virtue of the histopathology and immunophenotype, CD14/CD68/CD163/F13a/fascin, without CD1a/CD207 and with low (variable to absent) S100. Dermal lesions tend to involute slowly over time. JXG lesions of the skin can follow treatment of LCH and rarely, combined elements of both are present. *ECD* can have a dermal component with xanthomatous papules or orbital xanthelasma, but the diagnosis should not be suggested unless there are other features.[28] The presence of *BRAF* mutation, however, in a dermal JXG-type lesion in the correct context may raise concern for ECD.

RDD of the skin presents generally as a deep dermal mass lesion often with lymphoid follicles. The diagnosis is made by recognizing the characteristic RDD cells and confirming the immunophenotype with selective S100 and fascin immunostaining.[29–31] Emperipolesis may be less prominent than in lymph nodes and late lesions are fibrosing, obscuring the residual islands of RDD. The differential diagnosis is from the reticulohistiocytoma JXG variant, which is superficial in the skin, lacking the strong S100 staining.

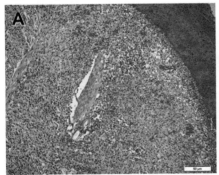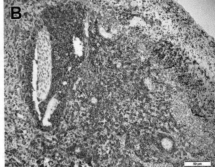

Fig. 4. (*A*) Papillary and reticular dermis infiltrated by LCH admixed with eosinophils and neutrophils with an overlying ulcerated epidermis. (*B*) The CD1a immunostain shows cytoplasmic granular staining. Original magnification ×200.

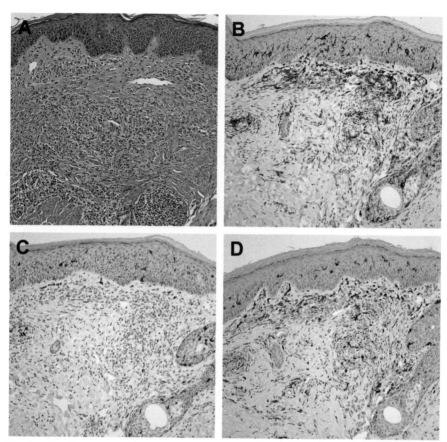

Fig. 5. (*A*) Subacute dermatitis, mostly superficial perivascular/periadnexal inflammatory cells with high content of histiocytes. (*B*) There is a perivascular distribution of spindly CD1a⁺ dermal histiocytes, in addition to the normal epidermal Langerhans cells. (*C*) CD207 highlights only the epidermal Langerhans cells. (*D*) S100 shows a similar distribution as CD1a. Original magnification ×200.

Lymph Nodes

LCH involvement in lymph nodes can be SS or part of MS disease. Patients present with asymptomatic localized lymphadenopathy. Histologic patterns vary but as a rule must contain a sinus element, highlighted with CD1a or CD207.[32,33] In cases of paracortical infiltration by LCH, the cells are larger and have less expression of CD1a/CD207 compared with the sinus infiltrate. Atypical examples of nodal LCH include a high content of osteoclast-type giant cells, necrosis, and hemosiderin with less CD207 (**Fig. 6**).

Late LCH of the lymph node may evolve to have no or very few CD1a⁺ cells, replaced by a xanthomatous macrophage infiltrate, no longer diagnosable as LCH. Of note, JXG does not typically involve the lymph nodes. Rare examples of nodal "JXG" with cytologic atypia raise a suspicion for histiocytic sarcoma.

Needle biopsy may be informative if the sinus nature of the LCH infiltrate can be demonstrated. Caution with fine-needle aspiration requires the understanding that (1) not all nodal LCH cells express CD1a/CD207 with the same intensity, (2) endogenous medullary sinus cells can express CD207, and (3) dermatopathic lymphadenopathy

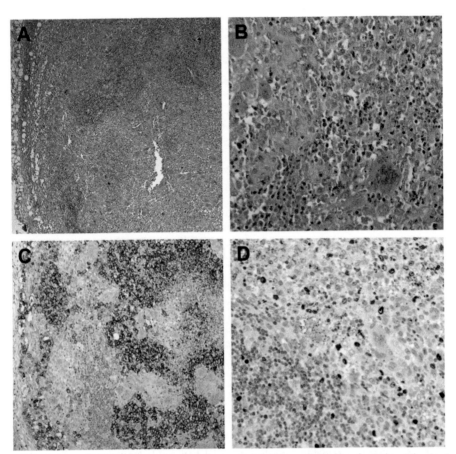

Fig. 6. (*A, B*) LCH infiltration with architectural distortion of the lymph node with giant cells, necrosis, and hemosiderin (H&E stain) (*A*, Original magnification ×200) (*B*, Original magnification ×400). (*C*) CD1a shows strong membranous staining of the LCH cells in the subcapsular sinus with infiltration into the paracortex (*C*, Original magnification ×200). (*D*) Ki-67 shows a mildly increased proliferation rate of the larger cells, taking into account background inflammatory cells (*D*, Original magnification ×400).

with high CD1a/CD207[+] population is excluded. Aspiration cytology may best be reserved for evaluating recurrence or disease extent rather than primary diagnosis.

There are no histologic features that predict systemic disease. Macrophage activation has been noted in nodes of multifocal and systemic disease, more commonly in young children with high-risk LCH and poor prognosis.[34] There is no significant difference in the proliferation rate between SS and MS disease but there have been no well-designed studies investigating dual CD207/Ki-67 expression. Ki-67 proliferation index is quoted to be from 2.6% to 48%,[35] although in our experience it is generally in the range of 10% or less in dual-stained cells.

An important differential diagnosis is with dermatopathic lymphadenopathy, which shows a nodular paracortical T-cell hyperplasia, expansion of S100[+]/fascin[+] interdigitating dendritic cells, paracortical CD1a[+]/CD207[+] Langerhans cells, along with macrophages containing melanin. The distinction from LCH includes the paracortical expansion, lack of sinus involvement, and high fascin positivity of the interdigitating dendritic cells (**Fig. 7**). Also it is important to use both CD1a and CD207 in the lymph node because there are endogenous CD207$^+$/CD1a$^-$ cells in the medullary sinuses.[10]

A differential diagnosis to consider especially in the adult is a primary Langerhans cell sarcoma. As a primary sarcoma, it is not preceded by LCH and has large, pleomorphic malignant cells with increased mitotic figures (more than 50 per 10 high power fields, Ki-67 >30%), many of which are atypical. The CD1a$^+$/CD207$^+$/S100$^+$ immunophenotype is preserved along with the sinus pattern. Expression of these markers can be variably lost with recurrences.

Other confounders in the lymph node are the histiocyte-rich variant of anaplastic large cell lymphoma, T-cell acute leukemia/lymphoma, granulomatous lymphadenitis, Churg-Strauss syndrome, and Kukuchi disease.

JXG and ECD rarely involve lymph nodes except by contiguous growth. RDD in the lymph node is the prototypical sinus histiocytosis with massive lymphadenopathy and relies on demonstrating the S100$^+$/fascin$^+$ RDD cells. There are examples of LCH and RDD in the same node or at different sites in the same patient (**Fig. 8**).

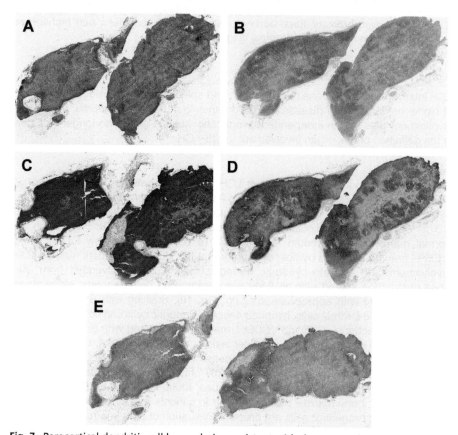

Fig. 7. Paracortical dendritic cell hyperplasia consistent with dermatopathic effect (*A*, H&E). The paracortical areas stain strongly with interdigitating cells (*B*, S100; *C*, Fascin). There is a high content of interspersed dendritic Langerhans cells (*D*, CD1a; *E*, CD207) in the expanded paracortex, without a sinus pattern. (Digital whole slide images (WSI) are hosted courtesy of University of Pittsburgh School of Medicine, Department of Pathology, Division of Informatics with permission.)

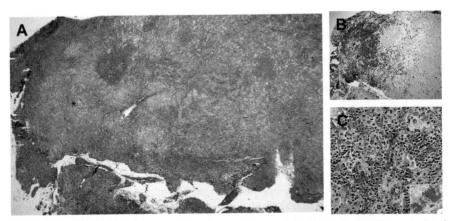

Fig. 8. (A) Mixed Rosai-Dorfman disease along with a nodule of LCH (*asterisk*) in an orbital lesion with lymphoid follicles and plasma cell–rich infiltrate (H&E stain) (Original magnification ×40). (B) CD1a immunostain highlights the LCH nodule (Original magnification ×20). (C) The large, hypochromatic Rosai-Dorfman cells display emperipolesis, best highlighted by the S100 immunostain (*inset*) (Original magnification ×400).

High-Risk Organ Involvement

LCH involvement of the bone marrow, liver, and spleen are considered to be markers of higher risk of dying of disease (ie, risk organs). In multivariate analysis, pulmonary involvement was not an independent prognostic variable and is no longer included in the definition of risk organ involvement in MS-LCH.[36]

Bone marrow

Although hematopoietic involvement in LCH is clinically defined by cytopenia of at least two cell lineages,[18] it is exceptional to find marrow replacement by LCH. Rather when present, there are only a few small clusters of CD1a+/CD207+ cells (<10–20 CD1a+ cells per slide) associated with more severe disease (**Fig. 9**).[37] Although the normal marrow biopsy should not have CD1a+/CD207+ cells, few CD1a+ cells (<0.5%) may be detected by flow cytometry, but this does not indicate marrow LCH involvement.[37] In aspirate cytology, distinguishing marrow involvement from lytic bone destruction should rest on finding accompanying hematopoietic elements in the former along with appropriate imaging (**Fig. 10**). Staining with S100 should be avoided because stromal cells, lymphocytes, and dendritic cells can confound.[38] Xanthomatous collections of CD163+/CD68+ macrophages along with areas of stromal fibrosis may be seen, particularly in older lesions or after treatment, but aggregates of macrophages are also seen in active disease without CD1a+/CD207+ histiocytes (**Fig. 11**). Conventionally, lack of CD1a+/CD207+ histiocytes is regarded as nondiagnostic for LCH. However, Berres and colleagues[8] found the BRAF V600E mutation in CD34+/CD207− bone marrow progenitor cells in patients with systemic disease indicating that LCH progenitor cells are present. Evaluation of bone marrow involvement with sensitive polymerase chain reaction methods for the detection of BRAF V600E is needed to better define hemopoietic involvement in LCH patients because CD1a and CD207 are not reliable markers in the bone marrow. Lastly, the marrow may also be populated with activated CD163+/CD68+ macrophages in cases of macrophage activation syndrome/hemophagocytic syndrome. The resultant cytokine storm is a possible underlying mechanism for cytopenias.[34,39]

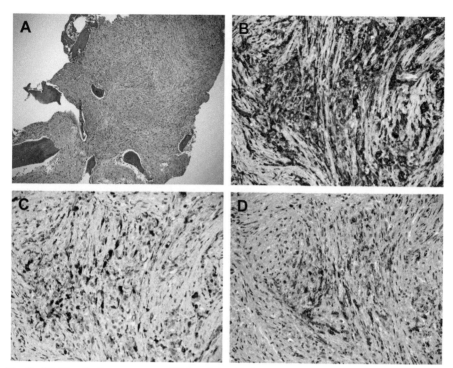

Fig. 9. (*A*) Fibrotic bone marrow (H&E stain) with (*B*) numerous CD163$^+$ macrophages and hemosiderin deposition. Scattered clusters of LCH cells, which although not morphologically distinguishable, are highlighted by (*C*) CD207 and (*D*) CD1a immunostains with a Prussian blue iron counterstain. (*A*, original magnification ×100; *B*, original magnification ×400; *C*, original magnification ×400; *D*, original magnification ×400).

JXG can involve the marrow as part of systemic disease, and is distinguished from LCH by histopathology, the lack of CD1a/CD207, and the presence of JXG markers.[40,41] Marrow failure and cytopenias are rare. ECD can involve the marrow with focal lesions but may be difficult to separate from bone involvement. RDD can involve the marrow when part of systemic disease, and the diagnostic findings are those of the RDD cell in a fibrosing lesion.

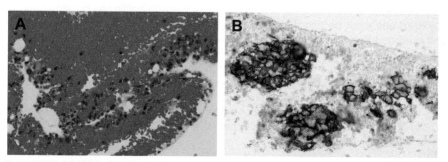

Fig. 10. (*A*) Cytology aspirate from a lytic lumbar spine lesion with LCH clusters admixed with blood; not a true bone marrow aspirate (H&E stain) (original magnification ×400). (*B*) The cell block preparation shows a cluster of CD1a$^+$ cells (original magnification ×400).

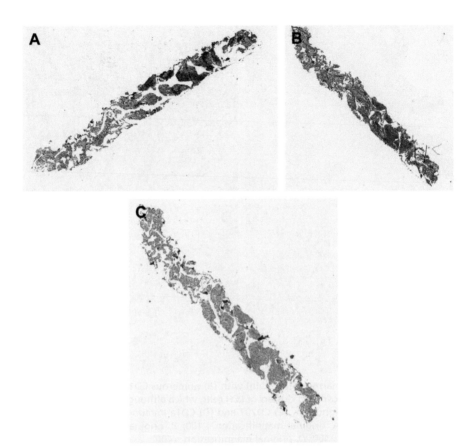

Fig. 11. History of a skin LCH diagnosed 2 months previously. The bone marrow shows cohesive sheets of macrophages, highlighted by (*A*) CD163 immunostain. The macrophages show (*B*) PAS-positive granular intracytoplasmic material. The bone marrow is nondiagnostic for LCH, in the absence of surface/membranous staining of (*C*) CD1a. (Digital whole slide images (WSI) are hosted courtesy of University of Pittsburgh School of Medicine, Department of Pathology, Division of Informatics with permission.)

Spleen

Clinical parameters define splenic LCH involvement by splenomegaly greater than 3 cm below the costal margin at the midclavicular line and confirmed by ultrasound[18]; however, one must be mindful that macrophage activation with hemophagocytosis and extramedullary hematopiesis can also cause splenic enlargement in the absence of true LCH involvement.[42] Splenic involvement confers a poor prognosis with more prolonged and intensive therapies.[18] When histologically confirmed, the LCH cells show sinus involvement.[35] Typically diagnosis is difficult to make on needle biopsy or aspiration cytology and is more commonly documented at splenectomy or autopsy. JXG is rarely a diagnostic consideration in the spleen, except in systemic disease.[43] ECD and RDD generally do not involve the spleen.

Liver

Liver involvement is more typically seen in the context of systemic LCH as compared with SS involvement.[44,45] Clinical involvement may be considered if there is enlargement greater than 3 cm below the costal margin at the midclavicular line; confirmed by ultrasound; or dysfunction documented by hyperbilirubinemia greater than three times normal, hypoalbuminemia (<30 g/dL), γ-glutamyltransferase (gGT) increased greater than two times normal, alanine aminotransferase or aspartate aminotransferase greater than three times normal, ascites, edema, or intrahepatic nodular masses. Liver biopsy is only recommended if there is clinically significant liver involvement or if the result alters treatment.[18] Histopathologic confirmation of putative hepatic LCH is required if there is no proven disease elsewhere. LCH is unique among the histiocytic disorders that involve the liver in that there is an exquisite tropism for the bile ducts leading to a destructive cholangiopathy and progression to biliary cirrhosis. Because LCH preferentially involves the large bile ducts (**Fig. 12**), it may be difficult to identify these changes on a liver biopsy (**Fig. 13**).[46] There is less involvement of the smaller peripheral interlobular ducts. The typical picture on liver biopsy is that of obstructive sclerosing cholangitis, uncommonly including sparse CD1a+/CD207+ LCH cells penetrating the basement membrane of bile ducts. However, because of the biliary tropism, when a diagnosis of LCH has been established elsewhere, a rising gGT and/or bilirubin with a histologic picture of sclerosing cholangitis is confirmatory of liver involvement, even in the absence of LCH cells.[44,45,47]

In MS-LCH disease, there may be hepatomegaly and hypoalbuminemia with a normal gGT or alkaline phosphatase levels. Such cases show no evidence of peribiliary LCH cells or sclerosing cholangitis but may display activated sinusoidal

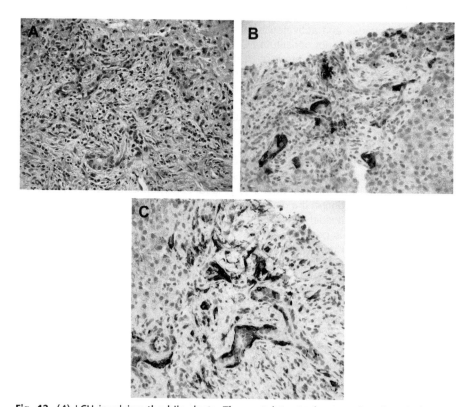

Fig. 12. (A) LCH involving the bile ducts. The portal tracts show a sclerosing cholangitis pattern with ductular proliferation and infiltration of the duct epithelium by (B) CD1a+ and (C) CD207+ cells, confirming the LCH infiltrate. Original magnification ×400.

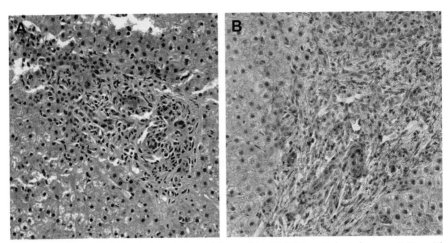

Fig. 13. (*A*) Liver biopsy from a 2-year-old boy with MS-LCH and ductular reactivity with pericholangitis (H&E stain). (*B*) CD1a immunostain is negative for LCH cells. Although the biopsy is nondiagnostic for LCH cells, the histologic findings together with an elevated gGT are highly suggestive of liver involvement. The patient went on to develop progressive liver disease with cirrhosis. Original magnification ×400.

CD68[+] macrophages and activated Kupffer cells, which can acquire S100-positivity.[34,47] This alone does not constitute LCH liver involvement.[34,47] In the later stages of the disease, the LCH infiltrate that destroys bile ducts can regress leaving only the resultant damage behind with biliary cirrhosis. This is a largely irreversible process that often results in the need for liver transplantation.[44] LCH recurrence in the liver allograft has been demonstrated in two pediatric MS-LCH cases,[48] along with a case of apparently de novo/primary MS-LCH (diagnosed from skin and lymph node involvement) occurring after living donor liver transplant for fulminant hepatic failure of unknown cause.[49]

JXG shows a portal expansion of bland oval nuclei and fairly abundant vacuolated and foamy cytoplasm and can also be associated with macrophage activation. The portal expansion, lack of bile duct injury, and immunophenotype (CD14/CD68/CD163/F13a/fascin) confirm the diagnosis (**Fig. 14**).[47]

RDD of the liver is unusual and in most instances accompanies systemic and nodal disease elsewhere. It is generally seen as nodules of RDD, diagnosed by the usual criteria. Hyperplastic Kupffer cells with hemophagocytosis can look similar. A sinus pattern of involvement has been seen in the RDD that accompanies the *SLC29A3* mutation with hepatosplenomegaly.[17]

Thymus

Much of the older literature describing the histologic patterns in thymus LCH was before the routine use of CD1a/CD207 and macrophages could not be reliably distinguished from LCH cells. Four distinct histologic patterns are seen in regards to thymic involvement.[50] Microscopic collection of Langerhans cells resembling LCH cells with round plump cytoplasm and nondendritic processes are seen in incidental thymectomies and myasthenia gravis thymectomies without LCH disease elsewhere. This group requires no further treatment and is thought to be a focal LCH-like hyperplasia with no clinical consequence.[50,51] In solitary and/or cystic SS-LCH of the thymus, there is architecture disruption with punctate calcifications, foci of necrosis, and a

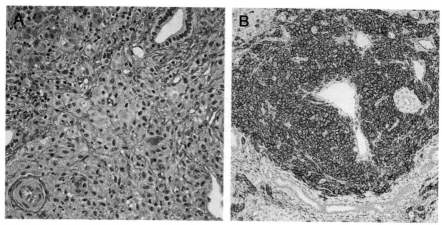

Fig. 14. (A) JXG infiltrate with a portal histiocytic infiltrate of plump histiocytes, occasional Touton-type giant cells, but no bile duct injury (H&E stain). The cells display a JXG immunophenotype including positivity for (B) CD163, and CD68/CD14/fascin/Factor 13a (not shown). (A, original magnification ×400; B, original magnification ×200).

variable fibrotic response.[50] The main differential diagnosis is mediastinal Hodgkin lymphoma. Confirmation of CD1a/CD207+ LCH cells, which are larger than CD1a+ cortical thymocytes, establishes the diagnosis. In MS-LCH, thymic involvement has a variable histologic pattern from medullary-restricted LCH infiltrates to diffuse gland involvement.[50] Thymic involvement may be missed at the time of LCH diagnosis if not directly imaged.[52,53] We have also seen two cases with a mixed histiocytic pattern with features of both LCH and a JXG-like proliferation in the thymus,[50] although solitary thymic JXG is unknown. RDD can occur in the mediastinum and very exceptionally, in the thymus as a nodular mass.

Thyroid

Like the thymus, LCH involvement can show variable manifestations in the thyroid. In MS-LCH, thyroid involvement may present as hypothyroidism and should be distinguished from hypothalamic-pituitary involvement. A goiter may be present in SS disease[54] or in MS disease.[55] Reported cases of thyroid LCH are more common in adults, especially as SS disease, but pediatric cases are seen in MS-LCH. There have also been reports of papillary thyroid carcinoma in patients who have MS-LCH.[56–59] Reports of concomitant clusters of CD1a/CD207+ Langerhans cells in a thyroid with papillary thyroid carcinoma may more likely represent LCH-like hyperplasia and not true LCH disease, similar to that described in lymph nodes and the thymus.[50,60] Because thyroid papillary thyroid carcinoma and LCH are known to share the same V600E point mutation in the BRAF gene, further investigation is needed to understand their molecular connection.[61]

JXG is not seen in the thyroid, although nodular involvement with ECD disease is described. RDD disease involving the thyroid is not that unusual even in the absence of systemic disease.

Lung

In children, lung involvement is seen in about a quarter of MS-LCH cases at diagnosis, but its impact on survival has been dismissed and is no longer considered a risk organ[18,36] In young adults 20 to 40 years old, LCH lung involvement is typically a single organ site and is closely associated with cigarette smoking, but can be seen in MS-LCH disease.[62–64] Although many cases are found incidentally, the bronchocentric involvement can lead to respiratory symptoms including dry cough and dyspnea, along with chest pain when associated with pneumothorax from subpleural cyst rupture. High-resolution computed tomography shows a bilateral symmetric bronchocentric process with centrilobular nodules in early lesions. As the lesions age, thin- and thick-walled cystic lesions are seen, evenly distributed between the central and peripheral portions of the upper and middle lobes.[62] Diagnosis is confirmed with CD1a/CD207+ LCH cells in the expected bronchocentric pattern.[63] Early lesions begin as a proliferation of LCH cells along the small airways and progress to bronchiolocentric nodules with extension into the alveolar septa (**Fig. 15**). A respiratory bronchiolitis caused by interstitial lung disease may masquerade with this pattern but is negative for CD1a/CD207+ LCH cells. As the lesion invades and destroys the bronchiolar walls, cavitary lesions may form. There is a mixed inflammatory infiltrate with pigmented alveolar macrophages, which may cause diagnostic confusion with desquamative interstitial pneumonia when extensive. Over time, the nodules become fibrotic and stellate scars with interstitial fibrosis produce permanent architectural disruption with honeycomb-like enlargement of the air spaces and hyperinflation. In older lesions, LCH cells may be absent making a definite diagnosis in the absence of disease elsewhere impossible. Bronchoalveolar lavage cytology with greater than 5% CD1a/CD207+ LCH may be used to diagnose LCH involvement in the appropriate clinical-radiographic context; however, it has low sensitivity.[65] Of note, smokers in general have an increased number of Langerhans cells, and their mere presence by staining does not indicate a pulmonary LCH lesion.[62] Thus the use of bronchoalveolar lavage cytology is heighted when combined with transbronchial biopsy in the appropriate clinicoradiographic setting.

In comparison with MS/multifocal LCH, adult localized disease may represent a reactive polyclonal process or even a hyperplastic response induced by the cigarette smoke in most cases.[66] However, recent molecular studies have shown the BRAF V600E mutation in 24% to 40% of adult pulmonary LCH, suggesting that a subset is clonal.[67,68] Recurrent pulmonary LCH after transplantation may occur in up to

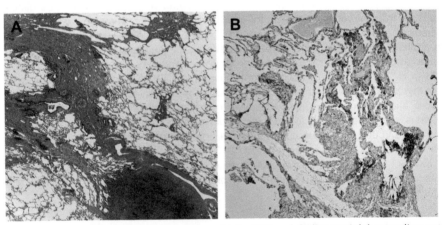

Fig. 15. (A) Lung with a large active peribronchiolar LCH nodule (*lower right*) extending out into the parenchyma, along with surrounding fibrosis and entrapped bronchiolar-associated lymphoid tissue (original magnification ×20). (B) CD1a immunostain highlights LCH aggregates around a small airway (original magnification ×100).

20% of cases, but does not seem to have significant impact on survival rate. Preoperative extrapulmonary LCH involvement and smoking recommencement are the main risk factors for recurrence in the graft.[69]

JXG of the lung is exceptional as a solitary mass, but can be seen in systemic disease. The lung, however, is a major site of predilection for ECD. ECD involves the lung in about 50% of patients and has a characteristic septal and subpleural pattern that produces MRI images of smooth interstitial thickening and cystic spaces, unlike LCH, which is peribronchial. Nodules are occasionally described. Diagnosis is usually suspected before biopsy, which is confirmatory when the histology is that of the JXG family or xanthomatous with an appropriate immunophenotype.[70] Intrathoracic RDD can include mediastinal lymphadenopathy and parenchymal disease without nodal involvement.[71] Some cases have been associated with IgG4 disease.[72,73]

Gastrointestinal Tract

The gastrointestinal tract is commonly involved in MS-LCH, and is often associated with high-risk disease and younger age (<2 year old). Gastrointestinal involvement can present as failure to thrive with diarrhea, bloody stools/anemia, vomiting, and protein-losing enteropathy.[74–76] Adult gastrointestinal involvement tends to be less ominous with few, if any, presenting features and overall better outcomes.[75] Polypoid mucosal lesions can be seen, and the differential diagnosis includes lymphoma and carcinoma in adult patients.[75,77,78] Site of involvement includes small bowel, colon, and stomach. On biopsy, there is a patchy to diffuse mucosal infiltration of CD1a/CD207+ LCH cells, which can extend into the submucosa. JXG involving the bowel is rare but ECD may rarely be a site of involvement.[79] RDD can involve the gastrointestinal tract, and some cases are associated with IgG4 disease.[80,81]

Central Nervous System

CNS involvement varies with a spectrum of cases ranging from (1) active LCH dominated by endocrine effects of pituitary and hypothalamic involvement; (2) spontaneous regression; (3) rapidly progressive to fatal disease; and (4) slow progressive neurodegenerative disease without LCH cells, which is thought to be a paraneoplastic process. DI is the most frequent endocrinopathy, resulting from LCH involvement of the neurohypophysis, which can present before, concurrently, or after a diagnosis of LCH.[18] Other endocrinopathies (eg, growth failure, precocious/delayed puberty, hypothyroidism, and so forth) may present if there is anterior pituitary involvement. SS-CNS involvement is described, but most cases occur in the context of MS disease with DI and associated "CNS-risk" craniofacial bone involvement (vide supra).[82,83]

Although neuroimaging has defined many patterns of LCH in the appropriate clinical setting, the neuropathology of LCH has been classified into three broad groups: (1) hypothalamic/pituitary axis involvement, (2) space-occupying CNS lesions, and (3) cerebellar/neurodegenerative lesions.[84] LCH involvement of the hypothalamic/pituitary axis is often seen in early, active disease with an infiltrating CD1a/CD207+ LCH population (**Fig. 16**). Of note, the general use of S100 immunostaining in the CNS is cautioned, given the extensive staining of endogenous CNS structures. Hypothalamic/pituitary axis involvement shows classic MRI findings, including infundibular thickening and lack of the posterior pituitary bright spot on T1-weighted images. Biopsy may be needed to establish a diagnosis in patients without evidence of LCH disease elsewhere. A variety of other diseases can cause infundibular thickening including germ cell tumors, sarcoidosis, tuberculosis, and nonspecific lymphocytic hypophysitis. Hypothalamic involvement may include glioma, lymphoma, hamartoma, and sarcoidosis.[84] The "granulomatous" infundibular LCH lesions may invade the

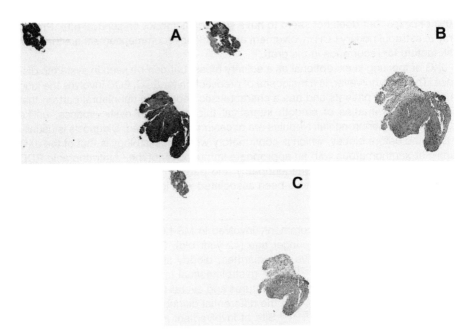

Fig. 16. A 10-year-old boy with DI and a hypothalamic tumor. (*A*) H&E shows numerous eosinophils with small numbers of LCH cells, highlighted by (*B*) CD1a surface and (*C*) CD207 cytoplasmic immunostaining. (Digital whole slide images (WSI) are hosted courtesy of University of Pittsburgh School of Medicine, Department of Pathology, Division of Informatics with permission.)

hypothalamus and surrounding CNS parenchyma with a CD8[+] T cell–rich inflammatory infiltrate and neurodegeneration with loss of axons and neurons.[85]

Space-occupying lesions often involve the leptomeninges, choroid plexus, and pineal gland with/without associated intraparenchymal involvement. Confined parenchymal involvement is less common and typically presents at a later age.[86] Symptoms depend on site and size of the lesion and are related to elevated intracerebral pressure and/or localized site of involvement (eg, headache, vomiting, papilledema, seizures). The histopathology of early lesions may show a CD1a/CD207[+] "granulomatous" LCH lesion with a surrounding T cell–rich inflammatory response. Older lesions typically show a fibroxanthomatous lesion with plump macrophages and Touton-type giant cells but few if any CD1a/CD207[+] LCH cells (**Fig. 17**). The latter finding can mimic a fibroxanthoma or JXG but does not typically express Factor 13a.[35] These lesions may represent regressed LCH (**Fig. 18**).[84]

The third group of CNS involvement includes neurologic degeneration, most commonly of the cerebellum, brainstem, and/or basal ganglia occurring years after a diagnosis of LCH. This process is thought to represent a paraneoplastic process with a T cell–rich inflammatory component with demyelination, loss of neurons and axons, but without CD1a/CD207[+] LCH cells.[85] This area is covered in more detail Ref.[87]

JXG can involve the spinal canal as solitary space-occupying lesions or as multiple lesions in more systemic disease.[88,89] There is some predilection for Meckel cave.[90] Most lesions are based on the meninges and only rarely are there intraparenchymal lesions. Despite their unusual and unexpected site, the histopathology and immunophenotype are quite typical and Touton cells may provide a clue. A rare lesion with

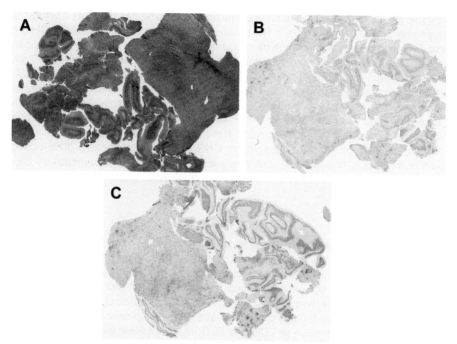

Fig. 17. A 24-year-old woman with a long history of MS-LCH diagnosed at the age of 2 years with high-risk CNS lesions and DI. Presented with obstructing hydrocephalus and heterogeneously enhancing cerebellar masses on MRI with mass effect on the fourth ventricle. (*A*) H&E shows architectural distortion of the cerebellum with a rich inflammatory infiltrate and very small nodules of LCH highlighted by (*B*) CD1a and (*C*) CD207). (Digital whole slide images (WSI) are hosted courtesy of University of Pittsburgh School of Medicine, Department of Pathology, Division of Informatics with permission.)

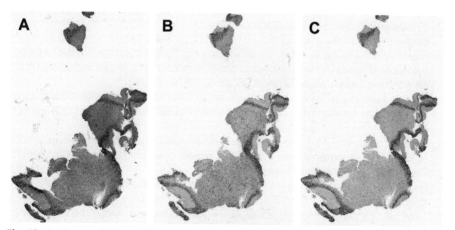

Fig. 18. A 15-year-old boy with a pineal mass and multiple cerebellar and brainstem lesions on MRI, along with a spinal lesion. The cerebellar (*A*) H&E and pineal biopsy (not scanned) showed a xanthomatous histiocytic infiltrate, highlighted by (*B*) CD68 immunostain, but there were no (*C*) CD1a+ LCH cells present. (Digital whole slide images (WSI) are hosted courtesy of University of Pittsburgh School of Medicine, Department of Pathology, Division of Informatics with permission.)

cytologic atypia, high turnover, and abnormal mitoses can be described as a histiocytic sarcoma with JXG phenotype.[12] The problem of lesions that follow treated LCH but have JXG morphology and phenotype has already been alluded to. ECD similarly can involve the CNS as part of more systemic disease but lesions confined to the CNS are also described.[91,92] ECD shares with LCH the capacity to involve the posterior pituitary not uncommonly causing DI. The diagnosis is established in general by the entire clinical, imaging, and histopathologic evidence. Solitary intracranial ECD presents a unique challenge. The presence of BRAF V600E mutation is helpful in establishing the correct diagnosis in a CNS lesion that has features of the JXG family.

Extranodal RDD can involve the spine or CNS, more commonly as a dural-based lesion mimicking a meningioma, but rarely as intracerebral or intramedullary disease.[93,94] The lesions are masses that have the diagnostic features of RDD.

SUMMARY

The classification of LCH will continue to be refined as more understanding into the bone marrow precursor is gained and its molecular pathogenesis is further understood. This will be especially useful in cases where the basic histopathology and immunophenotype are not clearly defined, as seen in older lesions with a "burnt-out" fibrotic appearance and in cases of mixed histiocytic disorders. Also further insight into the molecular biology of histiocytosis is revealing new evidence that previously separate lesions, such as LCH and ECD, share a similar molecular signature. This molecular awakening may help define lineage-specific markers that could better aid the diagnosis and classification of these more challenging histiocytic lesions. Thus as more is learned about the molecular biology of the histiocytoses, future classifications will be refined.

REFERENCES

1. Hervier B, Haroche J, Arnaud L, et al. Association of both Langerhans cell histiocytosis and Erdheim-Chester disease linked to the BRAFV600E mutation: a multicenter study of 23 cases. Blood 2014;124(7):1119–26.
2. O'Malley DP, Duong A, Barry TS, et al. Co-occurrence of Langerhans cell histiocytosis and Rosai-Dorfman disease: possible relationship of two histiocytic disorders in rare cases. Mod Pathol 2010;23(12):1616–23.
3. Abla O, Halliday W, Laughlin S, et al. Central nervous system juvenile xanthogranuloma after Langerhans cell histiocytosis. Pediatr Blood Cancer 2013;60(2): 342–3.
4. Bains A, Parham DM. Langerhans cell histiocytosis preceding the development of juvenile xanthogranuloma: a case and review of recent developments. Pediatr Dev Pathol 2011;14(6):480–4.
5. Rezk SA, Spagnolo DV, Brynes RK, et al. Indeterminate cell tumor: a rare dendritic neoplasm. Am J Surg Pathol 2008;32(12):1868–76.
6. Chan JK, Lamant L, Algar E, et al. ALK+ histiocytosis: a novel type of systemic histiocytic proliferative disorder of early infancy. Blood 2008;112(7):2965–8.
7. Badalian-Very G, Vergilio JA, Degar BA, et al. Recurrent BRAF mutations in Langerhans cell histiocytosis. Blood 2010;116(11):1919–23.
8. Berres ML, Lim KP, Peters T, et al. BRAF V600E expression in precursor versus differentiated dendritic cells defines clinically distinct LCH risk groups. J Exp Med 2014;211(4):669–83.

9. Lau SK, Chu PG, Weiss LM. Immunohistochemical expression of Langerin in Langerhans cell histiocytosis and non-Langerhans cell histiocytic disorders. Am J Surg Pathol 2008;32(4):615–9.
10. Chikwava K, Jaffe R. Langerin (CD207) staining in normal pediatric tissues, reactive lymph nodes, and childhood histiocytic disorders. Pediatr Dev Pathol 2004; 7(6):607–14.
11. Jaffe R, Chikwava K. Disorders of histiocytes. In: Hsi ED, editor. Hematopathology. 2nd edition. Philadelphia: Elsevier Saunders; 2012. p. 577.
12. Ernemann U, Skalej M, Hermisson M, et al. Primary cerebral non-Langerhans cell histiocytosis: MRI and differential diagnosis. Neuroradiology 2002;44(9):759–63.
13. Maric I, Pittaluga S, Dale JK, et al. Histologic features of sinus histiocytosis with massive lymphadenopathy in patients with autoimmune lymphoproliferative syndrome. Am J Surg Pathol 2005;29(7):903–11.
14. Maia DM, Dorfman RF. Focal changes of sinus histiocytosis with massive lymphadenopathy (Rosai-Dorfman disease) associated with nodular lymphocyte predominant Hodgkin's disease. Hum Pathol 1995;26(12):1378–82.
15. Delacretaz F, Meuge-Moraw C, Anwar D, et al. Sinus histiocytosis with massive lymphadenopathy (Rosai Dorfman disease) in an HIV-positive patient. Virchows Arch A Pathol Anat Histopathol 1991;419(3):251–4.
16. Menon MP, Evbuomwan MO, Rosai J, et al. A subset of Rosai-Dorfman disease cases show increased IgG4-positive plasma cells: another red herring or a true association with IgG4-related disease? Histopathology 2014;64(3):455–9.
17. Rossbach HC, Dalence C, Wynn T, et al. Faisalabad histiocytosis mimics Rosai-Dorfman disease: brothers with lymphadenopathy, intrauterine fractures, short stature, and sensorineural deafness. Pediatr Blood Cancer 2006;47(5):629–32.
18. Haupt R, Minkov M, Astigarraga I, et al. Langerhans cell histiocytosis (LCH): guidelines for diagnosis, clinical work-up, and treatment for patients till the age of 18 years. Pediatr Blood Cancer 2013;60(2):175–84.
19. Roncaroli F, Consales A, Galassi E, et al. Occipital aneurysmal bone cyst secondary to eosinophilic granuloma. Pediatr Neurosurg 2001;35(2):103–6.
20. Strehl JD, Stachel KD, Hartmann A, et al. Juvenile xanthogranuloma developing after treatment of Langerhans cell histiocytosis: case report and literature review. Int J Clin Exp Pathol 2012;5(7):720–5.
21. Haroche J, Charlotte F, Arnaud L, et al. High prevalence of BRAF V600E mutations in Erdheim-Chester disease but not in other non-Langerhans cell histiocytoses. Blood 2012;120(13):2700–3.
22. Hashimoto K, Bale GF, Hawkins HK, et al. Congenital self-healing reticulohistiocytosis (Hashimoto-Pritzker type). Int J Dermatol 1986;25(8):516–23.
23. Mandel VD, Ferrari C, Cesinaro AM, et al. Congenital "self-healing" Langerhans cell histiocytosis (Hashimoto-Pritzker disease): a report of two cases with the same cutaneous manifestations but different clinical course. J Dermatol 2014; 41(12):1098–101.
24. Jaffe R. Is there a role for histopathology in predicting the clinical outcome in congenital and infant Langerhans cell disease? Pediatr Blood Cancer 2009; 53(6):924–5.
25. Varga E, Korom I, Polyanka H, et al. BRAFV600E mutation in cutaneous lesions of patients with adult Langerhans cell histiocytosis. J Eur Acad Dermatol Venereol 2014;29(6):1205–11.
26. Edelbroek JR, Vermeer MH, Jansen PM, et al. Langerhans cell histiocytosis first presenting in the skin in adults: frequent association with a second haematological malignancy. Br J Dermatol 2012;167(6):1287–94.

27. Ozono S, Inada H, Nakagawa S, et al. Juvenile myelomonocytic leukemia characterized by cutaneous lesion containing Langerhans cell histiocytosis-like cells. Int J Hematol 2011;93(3):389–93.

28. Skinner M, Briant M, Morgan MB. Erdheim-Chester disease: a histiocytic disorder more than skin deep. Am J Dermatopathol 2011;33(2):e24–6.

29. Thawerani H, Sanchez RL, Rosai J, et al. The cutaneous manifestations of sinus histiocytosis with massive lymphadenopathy. Arch Dermatol 1978;114(2):191–7.

30. Frater JL, Maddox JS, Obadiah JM, et al. Cutaneous Rosai-Dorfman disease: comprehensive review of cases reported in the medical literature since 1990 and presentation of an illustrative case. J Cutan Med Surg 2006;10(6):281–90.

31. Wang KH, Chen WY, Liu HN, et al. Cutaneous Rosai-Dorfman disease: clinico-pathological profiles, spectrum and evolution of 21 lesions in six patients. Br J Dermatol 2006;154(2):277–86.

32. Favara BE, Steele A. Langerhans cell histiocytosis of lymph nodes: a morphological assessment of 43 biopsies. Pediatr Pathol Lab Med 1997;17(5):769–87.

33. Edelweiss M, Medeiros LJ, Suster S, et al. Lymph node involvement by Langerhans cell histiocytosis: a clinicopathologic and immunohistochemical study of 20 cases. Hum Pathol 2007;38(10):1463–9.

34. Favara BE, Jaffe R, Egeler RM. Macrophage activation and hemophagocytic syndrome in Langerhans cell histiocytosis: report of 30 cases. Pediatr Dev Pathol 2002;5(2):130–40.

35. Schmitz L, Favara BE. Nosology and pathology of Langerhans cell histiocytosis. Hematol Oncol Clin North Am 1998;12(2):221–46.

36. Ronceray L, Potschger U, Janka G, et al. Pulmonary involvement in pediatric-onset multisystem Langerhans cell histiocytosis: effect on course and outcome. J Pediatr 2012;161(1):129–33.e1–3.

37. Minkov M, Potschger U, Grois N, et al. Bone marrow assessment in Langerhans cell histiocytosis. Pediatr Blood Cancer 2007;49(5):694–8.

38. Shin SS, Sheibani K, Kezirian J, et al. Immunoarchitecture of normal human bone marrow: a study of frozen and fixed tissue sections. Hum Pathol 1992;23(6):686–94.

39. Galluzzo ML, Braier J, Rosenzweig SD, et al. Bone marrow findings at diagnosis in patients with multisystem Langerhans cell histiocytosis. Pediatr Dev Pathol 2010;13(2):101–6.

40. Chantranuwat C. Systemic form of juvenile xanthogranuloma: report of a case with liver and bone marrow involvement. Pediatr Dev Pathol 2004;7(6):646–8.

41. Kesserwan C, Boue DR, Kahwash SB. Isolated juvenile xanthogranuloma in the bone marrow: report of a case and review of the literature. Pediatr Dev Pathol 2007;10(2):161–4.

42. Christiansen EC, Ellwein M, Neglia JP. Splenomegaly unresponsive to standard and salvage chemotherapy in Langerhans cell histiocytosis: a case of extramedullary hematopoiesis. Pediatr Blood Cancer 2012;58(6):998–9.

43. Dehner LP. Juvenile xanthogranulomas in the first two decades of life: a clinicopathologic study of 174 cases with cutaneous and extracutaneous manifestations. Am J Surg Pathol 2003;27(5):579–93.

44. Kaplan KJ, Goodman ZD, Ishak KG. Liver involvement in Langerhans' cell histiocytosis: a study of nine cases. Mod Pathol 1999;12(4):370–8.

45. Favara BE. Histopathology of the liver in histiocytosis syndromes. Pediatr Pathol Lab Med 1996;16(3):413–33.

46. Meyer JS, De Camargo B. The role of radiology in the diagnosis and follow-up of Langerhans cell histiocytosis. Hematol Oncol Clin North Am 1998;12(2):307–26.

47. Jaffe R. Liver involvement in the histiocytic disorders of childhood. Pediatr Dev Pathol 2004;7(3):214–25.
48. Hadzic N, Pritchard J, Webb D, et al. Recurrence of Langerhans cell histiocytosis in the graft after pediatric liver transplantation. Transplantation 2000;70(5):815–9.
49. Honda R, Ohno Y, Iwasaki T, et al. Langerhans' cell histiocytosis after living donor liver transplantation: report of a case. Liver Transpl 2005;11(11):1435–8.
50. Picarsic J, Egeler RM, Chikwava K, et al. Histologic patterns of thymic involvement in Langerhans cell proliferations: a clinicopathologic study and review of the literature. Pediatr Dev Pathol 2015;18(2):127–38.
51. Gilcrease MZ, Rajan B, Ostrowski ML, et al. Localized thymic Langerhans' cell histiocytosis and its relationship with myasthenia gravis. Immunohistochemical, ultrastructural, and cytometric studies. Arch Pathol Lab Med 1997;121(2):134–8.
52. Lakatos K, Herbruggen H, Potschger U, et al. Radiological features of thymic Langerhans cell histiocytosis. Pediatr Blood Cancer 2013;60(11):E143–5.
53. Ducassou S, Seyrig F, Thomas C, et al. Thymus and mediastinal node involvement in childhood Langerhans cell histiocytosis: long-term follow-up from the French national cohort. Pediatr Blood Cancer 2013;60(11):1759–65.
54. Patten DK, Wani Z, Tolley N. Solitary Langerhans histiocytosis of the thyroid gland: a case report and literature review. Head Neck Pathol 2012;6(2):279–89.
55. Xia CX, Li R, Wang ZH, et al. A rare cause of goiter: Langerhans cell histiocytosis of the thyroid. Endocr J 2012;59(1):47–54.
56. Vergez S, Rouquette I, Ancey M, et al. Langerhans cell histiocytosis of the thyroid is a rare entity, but an association with a papillary thyroid carcinoma is often described. Endocr Pathol 2010;21(4):274–6.
57. Jamaati HR, Shadmehr MB, Saidi B, et al. Langerhans cell histiocytosis of the lung and thyroid, co-existing with papillary thyroid cancer. Endocr Pathol 2009; 20(2):133–6.
58. Goldstein N, Layfield LJ. Thyromegaly secondary to simultaneous papillary carcinoma and histiocytosis X. Report of a case and review of the literature. Acta Cytol 1991;35(4):422–6.
59. Burnett A, Carney D, Mukhopadhyay S, et al. Thyroid involvement with Langerhans cell histiocytosis in a 3-year-old male. Pediatr Blood Cancer 2008;50(3): 726–7.
60. Christie LJ, Evans AT, Bray SE, et al. Lesions resembling Langerhans cell histiocytosis in association with other lymphoproliferative disorders: a reactive or neoplastic phenomenon? Hum Pathol 2006;37(1):32–9.
61. Moschovi M, Adamaki M, Vlahopoulos S, et al. Synchronous and metachronous thyroid cancer in relation to Langerhans cell histiocytosis; involvement of V600E BRAF-mutation? Pediatr Blood Cancer 2015;62(1):173–4.
62. Tazi A, Soler P, Hance AJ. Adult pulmonary Langerhans' cell histiocytosis. Thorax 2000;55(5):405–16.
63. Vassallo R, Ryu JH, Colby TV, et al. Pulmonary Langerhans'-cell histiocytosis. N Engl J Med 2000;342(26):1969–78.
64. Arico M, Girschikofsky M, Genereau T, et al. Langerhans cell histiocytosis in adults. Report from the International Registry of the Histiocyte Society. Eur J Cancer 2003;39(16):2341–8.
65. Baqir M, Vassallo R, Maldonado F, et al. Utility of bronchoscopy in pulmonary Langerhans cell histiocytosis. J Bronchology Interv Pulmonol 2013;20(4):309–12.
66. Dacic S, Trusky C, Bakker A, et al. Genotypic analysis of pulmonary Langerhans cell histiocytosis. Hum Pathol 2003;34(12):1345–9.

67. Yousem SA, Dacic S, Nikiforov YE, et al. Pulmonary Langerhans cell histiocytosis: profiling of multifocal tumors using next-generation sequencing identifies concordant occurrence of BRAF V600E mutations. Chest 2013;143(6):1679–84.

68. Roden AC, Hu X, Kip S, et al. BRAF V600E expression in Langerhans cell histiocytosis: clinical and immunohistochemical study on 25 pulmonary and 54 extrapulmonary cases. Am J Surg Pathol 2014;38(4):548–51.

69. Dauriat G, Mal H, Thabut G, et al. Lung transplantation for pulmonary langerhans' cell histiocytosis: a multicenter analysis. Transplantation 2006;81(5):746–50.

70. Arnaud L, Pierre I, Beigelman-Aubry C, et al. Pulmonary involvement in Erdheim-Chester disease: a single-center study of thirty-four patients and a review of the literature. Arthritis Rheum 2010;62(11):3504–12.

71. Cartin-Ceba R, Golbin JM, Yi ES, et al. Intrathoracic manifestations of Rosai-Dorfman disease. Respir Med 2010;104(9):1344–9.

72. Park BH, Son da H, Kim MH, et al. Rosai-Dorfman disease: report of a case associated with IgG4-related sclerotic lesions. Korean J Pathol 2012;46(6):583–6.

73. El-Kersh K, Perez RL, Guardiola J. Pulmonary IgG4+ Rosai-Dorfman disease. BMJ Case Rep 2013;2013.

74. Geissmann F, Thomas C, Emile JF, et al. Digestive tract involvement in Langerhans cell histiocytosis. The French Langerhans Cell Histiocytosis Study Group. J Pediatr 1996;129(6):836–45.

75. Singhi AD, Montgomery EA. Gastrointestinal tract Langerhans cell histiocytosis: a clinicopathologic study of 12 patients. Am J Surg Pathol 2011;35(2):305–10.

76. Shima H, Takahashi T, Shimada H. Protein-losing enteropathy caused by gastrointestinal tract-involved Langerhans cell histiocytosis. Pediatrics 2010;125(2): e426–32.

77. Groisman GM, Rosh JR, Harpaz N. Langerhans cell histiocytosis of the stomach. A cause of granulomatous gastritis and gastric polyposis. Arch Pathol Lab Med 1994;118(12):1232–5.

78. Iwafuchi M, Watanabe H, Shiratsuka M. Primary benign histiocytosis X of the stomach. A report of a case showing spontaneous remission after 5 1/2 years. Am J Surg Pathol 1990;14(5):489–96.

79. Detlefsen S, Fagerberg CR, Ousager LB, et al. Histiocytic disorders of the gastrointestinal tract. Hum Pathol 2013;44(5):683–96.

80. Anders RA, Keith JN, Hart J. Rosai-Dorfman disease presenting in the gastrointestinal tract. Arch Pathol Lab Med 2003;127(2):E74–5.

81. Wimmer DB, Ro JY, Lewis A, et al. Extranodal Rosai-Dorfman disease associated with increased numbers of immunoglobulin g4 plasma cells involving the colon: case report with literature review. Arch Pathol Lab Med 2013;137(7):999–1004.

82. Morimoto A, Ishida Y, Suzuki N, et al. Nationwide survey of single-system single site Langerhans cell histiocytosis in Japan. Pediatr Blood Cancer 2010;54(1): 98–102.

83. Gadner H, Heitger A, Grois N, et al. Treatment strategy for disseminated Langerhans cell histiocytosis. DAL HX-83 Study Group. Med Pediatr Oncol 1994;23(2): 72–80.

84. Grois NG, Favara BE, Mostbeck GH, et al. Central nervous system disease in Langerhans cell histiocytosis. Hematol Oncol Clin North Am 1998;12(2):287–305.

85. Grois N, Fahrner B, Arceci RJ, et al. Central nervous system disease in Langerhans cell histiocytosis. J Pediatr 2010;156(6):873–81, 881.e1.

86. Hund E, Steiner H, Jansen O, et al. Treatment of cerebral Langerhans cell histiocytosis. J Neurol Sci 1999;171(2):145–52.

87. Neurodegeneration in LCH, in press.

88. Meshkini A, Shahzadi S, Zali A, et al. Systemic juvenile xanthogranuloma with multiple central nervous system lesions. J Cancer Res Ther 2012;8(2):311–3.
89. Deisch JK, Patel R, Koral K, et al. Juvenile xanthogranulomas of the nervous system: a report of two cases and review of the literature. Neuropathology 2013; 33(1):39–46.
90. Paulus W, Kirchner T, Michaela M, et al. Histiocytic tumor of Meckel's cave. An intracranial equivalent of juvenile xanthogranuloma of the skin. Am J Surg Pathol 1992;16(1):76–83.
91. Arnaud L, Hervier B, Neel A, et al. CNS involvement and treatment with interferon-alpha are independent prognostic factors in Erdheim-Chester disease: a multicenter survival analysis of 53 patients. Blood 2011;117(10):2778–82.
92. Jain RS, Sannegowda RB, Jain R, et al. Erdheim-Chester disease with isolated craniocerebral involvement. BMJ Case Rep 2013;2013.
93. Adeleye AO, Amir G, Fraifeld S, et al. Diagnosis and management of Rosai-Dorfman disease involving the central nervous system. Neurol Res 2010;32(6): 572–8.
94. Fukushima T, Yachi K, Ogino A, et al. Isolated intracranial Rosai-Dorfman disease without dural attachment: case report. Neurol Med Chir (Tokyo) 2011;51(2): 136–40.

Cell(s) of Origin of Langerhans Cell Histiocytosis

Matthew Collin, MD, PhD[a], Venetia Bigley, MD, PhD[a],
Kenneth L. McClain, MD, PhD[b], Carl E. Allen, MD, PhD[b],*

KEYWORDS

- Langerhans cell histiocytosis • BRAF • MAPK signaling • Dendritic cell
- Myeloid differentiation

KEY POINTS

- Dendritic cells (DCs) are immune cells that arise from different lineages with a shared function of presenting antigen and activating adaptive immunity.
- Langerhans cell histiocytosis (LCH) arises from myeloid DC precursors. Mitogen-activated protein kinase (MAPK) activation is a universal feature of CD1a⁺ langerin⁺ LCH cells. The clinical extent of LCH is related to the stage of development in which somatic MAPK mutations arise, either self-renewing progenitors or committed precursors.
- Activating MAPK mutations in hematopoietic stem cells and committed myeloid precursors support classification of LCH as a myeloid neoplasia.

INTRODUCTION TO LANGERHANS CELL HISTIOCYTOSIS
The Histiocytoses

The spectrum of histiocytic diseases is characterized by collections of abnormal histiocytes or, literally, tissue cells related to myeloid cells of the mononuclear phagocyte system (MPS).[1–4] LCH is defined by the presence of a large pale-staining histiocyte

The Texas Children's Cancer Center Histiocytosis Program (C.E. Allen and K.L. McClain) is supported by the HistioCure Foundation. Grant support includes NIH R01 (CA154489) (C.E. Allen and K.L. McClain), NIH SPORE in Lymphoma (P50CA126752) (C.E. Allen), and the St. Baldrick's Consortium Grant for the North American Consortium for Histiocytosis Research (C.E. Allen and K.L. McClain). M. Collin is supported by the Histiocytosis Research Trust (UK), the Leventis Foundation, and the Histiocytosis Association. V. Bigley is a Wellcome Trust Intermediate Fellow (WT088555MA).
The authors have no conflicting financial interests.
[a] Human Dendritic Cell Laboratory, Institute of Cellular Medicine, Newcastle University, Framlington Place, Newcastle upon Tyne NE2 4HH, UK; [b] Texas Children's Cancer Center, Baylor College of Medicine, One Baylor Plaza, Houston, TX 77030, USA
* Corresponding author. Feigin Research Center, 1102 Bates Street, Houston, TX 77030.
E-mail address: ceallen@txch.org

with high expression of CD1a and langerin (CD207) and containing Birbeck granules (**Fig. 1**). These features, shared with Langerhans cells (LCs) of the epidermis, are the basis of classifying the disease as an LCH. Prior to this, LCH was known as histiocytosis X, a disease entity incorporating historically described syndromes: Hand-Schüller-Christian disease, characterized by lytic bone lesions and mucosal lesions; Letterer-Siwe disease, a fatal hepatosplenomegaly; and eosinophilic granuloma of bone. The discovery of the Birbeck granule in LCs in 1961 and identification of the same organelle in histiocytosis X by Nezelof and colleagues[5] in 1965 formed the basis for modern models of LCH. Another influence driving this model of LCH at the same time was the model of the MPS in which peripheral macrophages were thought to be continually renewed from bone marrow–derived monocytes.[1] LCs had recently joined the MPS by virtue of their expression of MHC class II, complement and Fc receptors, and repopulation by bone marrow–derived cells after transplantation. The formation of LCH was, therefore, perceived to be an aberration of this development, leading to the accumulation of abnormal LC-like cells in inappropriate locations.

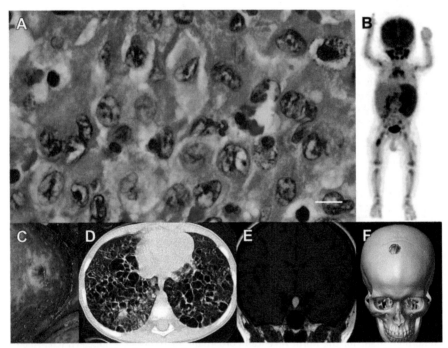

Fig. 1. LCH: common histology and clinical heterogeneity. (*A*) Hematoxylin-eosin staining of a typical LCH lesion, demonstrating the classic large histiocytes with grooved coffee bean nuclei and abundant eosinophilic cytoplasm. The inflammatory infiltrate varies but typically includes lymphocytes, eosinophils, and macrophages. Histologic features have not been associated with specific clinical presentations. Scale bar is 10 microns. (*B–F*) This biopsy could have come from any of the cases presented. (*B*) PET scan of a 1 year old with high-risk LCH: PET-avid R femur lesion, spleen, bone marrow, and cervical lymph nodes are evident in this image. (*C*) Infant with severe LCH skin lesions. In infants, skin LCH may be self-limiting and spontaneously resolve or may be part of life-threatening, multisystem, high-risk disease. (*D*) CT scan demonstrating innumerable cysts and lung lesions in a 3 year old with LCH involving lung, pituitary, and skin. (*E*) Brain MRI in a teenager with an isolated pituitary LCH lesion. (*F*) CT scan of a teenager with an isolated skull LCH lesion.

Clinical Overview

The clinical spectrum of LCH ranges from a trivial single lesion to aggressive and potentially lethal disseminated disease (see **Fig. 1**). Almost every organ system has been reported to be involved by LCH lesions. In infants, skin lesions are common and may represent skin-limited disease that resolves without therapy; alternatively, skin rash may be part of a constellation of lesions in disseminated multisystem disease. In older children and adults, presenting symptoms may include pain from bone lesions, dyspnea from lung lesions, failure to thrive from intestinal involvement, or uncontrolled thirst from pituitary infiltration and resulting diabetes insipidus. The range of presenting symptoms and overlapping clinical features with more common childhood conditions make LCH a challenging diagnosis. Once biopsy is performed, however, the unique features of LCH cells and the inflammatory context of lymphocytes, eosinophils, and macrophages are pathognomonic. Although the number of pathologic histiocytes and relative contribution of infiltrating leukocyte populations may be variable, the overall pattern is conserved across the spectrum of clinical manifestations of LCH (see **Fig. 1**).

Rationale for Current Approaches to Langerhans Cell Histiocytosis

Clinically, LCH has been categorized as having a high risk of mortality when it involves bone marrow, spleen, or liver or as low risk in any other site. Treatment regimens are empiric, as summarized by Arceci and colleagues[6] in the last *Hematology/Oncology Clinics of North America* issue dedicated to LCH (1998): "The variety of different treatment approaches to such patients has prompted some individuals to believe that LCH treatment 'strategy' is based more on a roulette wheel than on scientifically based logic. Certainly, part of the confusion and lack of consensus is derived from a persisting ambivalence as to whether LCH is primarily a neoplastic disorder, an immunodysrgulatory disorder, or a disorder with characteristics of both." Vinblastine and prednisone have been the standard induction therapy for decades, although LCH-II and LCH-III trials demonstrated improved outcomes with dose intensification and therapy prolongation.[7,8]

MOLECULAR INSIGHTS INTO PATHOGENESIS OF LANGERHANS CELL HISTIOCYTOSIS
Langerhans Cell Histiocytosis: The Debate

The fundamental nature of LCH as neoplastic versus reactive disorder has been an ongoing debate.[6,9] The granulomatous histology with quiescent histiocytes suggested potential autoimmune or infectious etiology[10] but the unique appearance of LCH cells and destructive nature of lesions hinted at dysplastic development. Although Nezelof and Basset[11] described LCs as the stem cell of LCH, they also acknowledged the prevailing view that elements of the MPS, including LCs, were continually replenished by the differentiation of bone marrow–derived precursors. Many hypotheses emerged that LCH might arise from LC precursors in a state of arrested development, misguided to inappropriate sites by a pathologic cytokine, or chemokine milieu,[12–14] but no unifying extrinsic explanation for pathologic LCH cell differentiation was ever achieved (reviewed by Laman and colleagues[15]). A neoplastic origin for LCH was suggested by the coincidence of LCH with myelodysplastic syndrome and other malignancies[16,17] and a major breakthrough came with the finding the LCH cells are clonal.[18,19] Persistent failure to identify genetic abnormalities in systematic analysis of LCH lesions, however, tempered classification of LCH as a cancer.[20–23]

Somatic Mitogen-Activated Protein Kinase Mutations in Langerhans Cell Histiocytosis

In 2010, Rollins and colleagues[24] reported the seminal finding of recurrent BRAF V600E point mutations in approximately 60% of LCH lesions. BRAF is a central kinase that transduces signals through the MAPK pathway, which regulates numerous essential cellular functions (**Fig. 2**A). The *BRAF* mutation encoding the V600E substitution leads to constitutive activation of downstream mitogen-activated protein kinase kinase (MEK) and extracellular signal-related kinase (ERK)[25] and is observed at high frequency in melanoma, in approximately 7% of human cancers overall, and in several benign neoplastic conditions, including epidermal nevi and colon polyps.[26,27] Subsequently, whole-exome sequencing of LCH lesions has revealed recurrent mutations in *MAP2K1* (encoding MEK1) in another 20% of patients and cases of mutations in other MAPK pathway genes, *ARAF* and *ERBB3*, on a low overall mutation rate background (0.03 mutations per megabase) (see **Fig. 2**).[28–30] These mutations all induce ERK activation, a universal feature of LCH cells.[24,29] The genomic landscape of LCH is discussed in detail elsewhere in this issue.[31]

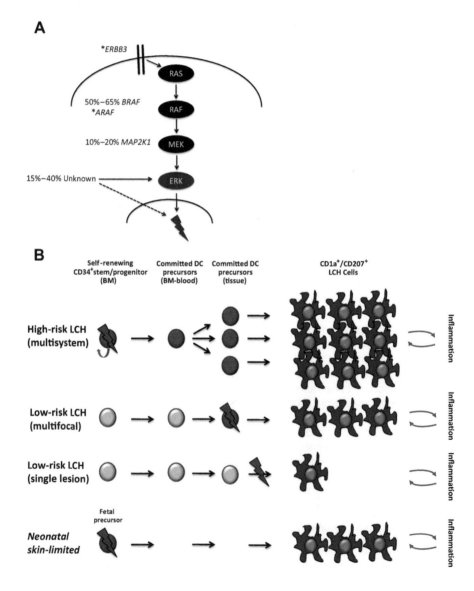

BRANCHES OF DENDRITIC CELL DIFFERENTIATION

The insight of Nezelof and Basset[32] identified commonality between LCs and LCH but by their own reckoning could not fully explain the histogenesis of LCH. The identification of MAPK pathway mutations provides a genetic neoplastic etiology and an important investigational tool with which to track potential LCH precursor cells. The problem of understanding exactly how potential LCH precursors differentiate abnormally remains, however, unsolved.

The Phenotype of Langerhans Cell Histiocytosis Dendritic Cells

To understand how aberrant DC differentiation might give rise to LCH cells, it is necessary to consider the phenotype of LCH cells in more detail. Breathnach and colleagues[33] noted that in addition to Birbeck granules, acid phosphatase, nonspecific esterase, and α-D mannosidase were expressed by LCs and LCH cells.[5] The advent of monoclonal OKT6, binding CD1a was a major advance both conceptually and diagnostically as was the description of langerin.[34] Expression of CD1a is universal in LCH, and typically CD1a and langerin are highly coexpressed. Birbeck granules are associated with high CD1a and langerin and are most abundant in the skin but may be absent in the liver and in old xanthomatous lesions.[35] Similarly, several reports describe heterogeneous states of differentiation of LCH cells within lesions, including variable CD1a+/langerin subpopulations.[35–37] Antibody-recognizing BRAF V600E (VE1) has also demonstrated that the mutation is present in some langerin− cells within LCH lesions.[38]

Despite these similarities, gene expression studies have demonstrated many differences between LCH cells and LCs: LCH cells express relatively less epithelial cell adhesion molecule (EpCAM), epithelial (E)-cadherin, and CD36; they also express higher levels of CD2, CD11b, CD11c, CD13, CD33, CD66c, and CD300LF, markers associated with myeloid DCs at all states of maturation. LCH cells also express high levels of cytokines and chemokines, including SPP1 (osteopontin), together with receptors CCR1 and NRP1 that influence capacity to recruit and interact with

◀───────────────────────────────

Fig. 2. Model of LCH pathogenesis: ERK activation at specific stages of myelopoiesis determines clinical phenotype. (*A*) Mutually exclusive activating mutations in MAPK genes have been reported in most cases of LCH, and ERK activation seems universal in LCH lesion CD207+ cells. Lightning bolt represents the downstream impact of ERK activation that presumably is essential for LCH pathogenesis. Astericks (*) indicates genes with case reports of mutations in LCH lesions. (*B*) Proposed misguided myeloid DC model of LCH pathogenesis in which somatic mutation (lightning bolt) and subsequent ERK activation (red cell) at specific stages of DC development determines clinical outcome. This model reflects interpretation of data from human and mouse studies[77] but leaves room for future refinement. According to this model, ERK activation in a self-renewing progenitor/stem cell in the bone marrow has the potential to form lesions in hematopoietic organs, liver, and virtually any organ system leading to MS LCH, with somatic mutation detectable in bone marrow (BM) and blood. In contrast, ERK activation in committed precursors may form multiple lesions in a limited number of organ systems, but somatic mutation is not usually detectable in the BM or blood at diagnosis or subsequently. ERK activation at a later stages of differentiation, perhaps even in a single tissue cell, may form a single unifocal lesion. Based on recent data describing the prenatal origin of tissue myeloid cells, it is also conceivable that ERK-activating mutation may arise during fetal development. This is speculative but could explain self-resolving neonatal LCH (Hashimoto-Pritzker syndrome) in which mutated fetal precursors are replaced by normal myeloid cells after birth. In all models, it is suggested that LCH cells recruit and activate inflammatory cells, which may provide reciprocal survival signals and clearly play a role in clinical manifestations of LCH. (*Data from* Refs.[28–30,77])

T cells.[39] When isolated from lesions, they are somewhat immature, promoting a T_H2-rich environment enriched with eosinophils and regulatory T cells.[21] These observations support a hypothesis that aberrant differentiation of a myeloid progenitor leads to a series of LC-like differentiation steps that are time and location dependent. The nature of this precursor remains undefined although the low expression of S100A8/9 indicates that LCH cells are unlikely to be recently derived from monocytes.[39]

Origin and Homeostasis of Langerhans Cells in the Steady State

It is now appreciated that LCs are unique not only in their residence in the epidermis and mucosae but also in their origin and homeostasis.[40] Contrary to the MPS model, LCs are not continually replenished from blood-borne progenitors in the steady state. The first LCs are derived from myeloid precursors during fetal life,[41,42] which differentiate under the influence of the colony stimulating factor 1 receptor (CSF1R) cytokine interleukin (IL)-34[43,44] and autocrine production of transforming growth factor (TGF)-β.[45] Ultimately, fetal LC progenitors are derived from primitive waves of hematopoiesis that are c-myb and flt3 independent and precede definitive hematopoiesis in the fetal liver.[46–48] Once seeded in the epidermis, LCs are able to undergo homeostatic self-renewal, as first suggested in humans[49] and proved by elegant experiments in mice.[22] The independence of LCs from monocytes and blood DCs in the steady state is also demonstrated by the preservation of these cells in patients with genetic deficiency of monocytes and DCs[50,51] and in patients who have received limb transplants.[52] The development and subsequent self-renewing potential of a tissue macrophage/DC network during fetal life raises new possibilities for the origin of LCH cells. It is conceivable that somatic mutation could arise in these cycling cells and could result in LCH or that activation of a more widely distributed fetal precursor could occur (see **Fig. 2B**).

Replenishment of Langerhans Cells During Inflammation

Although fetal-derived LCs are self-renewing in epidermis during steady state, bone marrow–derived precursors are recruited during inflammation, such as graft-vs-host disease after human stem cell transplantation.[53,54] In mice, the epidermis is initially infiltrated by classical monocytes,[55] but a second wave of more long-lived LC precursors has recently been described.[56,57] In a recapitulation of embryonic development, IL-34 is also required to maintain long-term LC repopulation.[56]

Dual Inflammatory Langerhans Cell Precursors

The duality of inflammatory LC precursors in mice also finds resonance with in vitro experiments in humans. A 2-phase kinetic was observed many years ago in serial skin biopsies of delayed-type hypersensitivity reactions.[58] Langerin+ cells can be derived from monocytes,[59–61] from CD14+ cells appearing in CD34+ cultures,[62] and from dermal CD14+ cells that are now known to be monocyte derived.[63,64] All these may represent the monocyte pathway of short-term recruitment. In addition, CD1a+ CD14− intermediates with restricted LC potential can be generated from CD34+ progenitors.[65,66] This suggests potential for an alternative pathway of LC differentiation, a conclusion that was recently supported by direct comparisons of CD14 monocytes and CD1c+ blood DCs exposed to LC differentiation conditions. In these experiments, surprisingly, CD1c+ DCs expressed much higher levels of CD1a and langerin than monocytes and only CD1c+ DCs rapidly formed Birbeck granules.[67,68] Either granulocyte-macrophage colony-stimulating factor or thymic stromal lymphopoietin was able to induce CD1a expression, and high langerin was promoted by TGF-β or bone morphogenetic protein 7. The role of IL-34 was not explored.

Together these results suggest that the DC differentiation pathway may contribute to long-term LC precursors observed in mice and, furthermore, that both bone marrow–derived monocytes and myeloid DCs can express langerin and are candidate precursors for LCH cells.

Langerhans Cells Are Not the Only Fruit: Other Human Dendritic Cells

LCs are the paradigmatic migratory DCs, but blood and interstitial tissues contain 2 other populations of myeloid DCs: a minor subset of CD141[+] cells and a major subset of CD1c[+] cells[69–71] (**Fig. 3**). Representatives of both are found in the blood and lymph nodes and are evolutionarily conserved in mammals, corresponding to the 2 subsets of classical or conventional DCs described in mice.[2,4] The term, *myeloid*, is specific in humans and refers to the expression of antigens typically seen on granulocytes or monocytes, including CD13, CD33, CD11b, and CD11c. Plasmacytoid DCs typically lack myeloid antigens and are morphologically and functionally distinct, providing a major source of type 1 interferon in response to viral infection (reviewed by Reizis and colleagues[72]). They are typically found only in lymph nodes and inflamed tissues. In addition, several monocyte-derived DCs and macrophages are found in human tissues.[63,73,74]

Langerin-Positive Dendritic Cells

It is now known that other DC lineage cells expression langerin. A small population of CD1c[+] DCs (the major myeloid DC), distinct from LCs and from CD141[+] DCs,

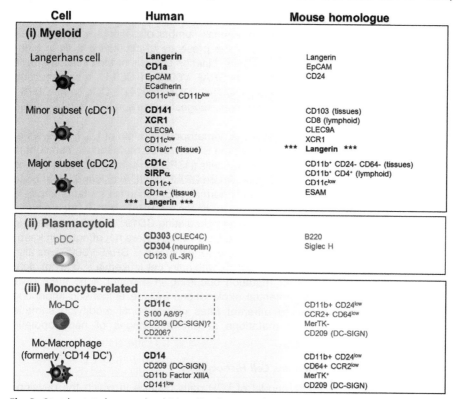

Cell	Human	Mouse homologue
(i) Myeloid		
Langerhans cell	**Langerin** **CD1a** EpCAM ECadherin CD11c[low] CD11b[low]	Langerin EpCAM CD24
Minor subset (cDC1)	**CD141** **XCR1** CLEC9A CD11c[low] CD1a/c[+] (tissue)	CD103 (tissues) CD8 (lymphoid) CLEC9A XCR1 *** **Langerin** ***
Major subset (cDC2)	**CD1c** **SIRPα** CD11c+ CD1a+ (tissue) *** **Langerin** ***	CD11b[+] CD24- CD64- (tissues) CD11b[+] CD4[+] (lymphoid) CD11c[low] ESAM
(ii) Plasmacytoid		
pDC	**CD303** (CLEC4C) **CD304** (neuropilin) CD123 (IL-3R)	B220 Siglec H
(iii) Monocyte-related		
Mo-DC	**CD11c** S100 A8/9? CD209 (DC-SIGN)? CD206?	CD11b+ CD24[low] CCR2+ CD64[low] MerTK- CD209 (DC-SIGN)
Mo-Macrophage (formerly 'CD14 DC')	**CD14** CD209 (DC-SIGN) CD11b Factor XIIIA CD141[low]	CD11b+ CD24[low] CD64+ CCR2[low] MerTK[+] CD209 (DC-SIGN)

Fig. 3. Steady-state human dendritic cells. The astericks in this case highlight cells other than conventional LCs with the ability to express Langerin.

expresses a low level of langerin in vivo.[70,75] Confusingly, langerin is also found on mouse DCs but restricted to the minor classical DC population, which is not the direct homologue of human CD1c$^+$ DCs[76] (see **Fig. 3**). The presence of langerin$^+$ CD1c$^+$ DCs in human tissues is consistent with the ability of blood CD1c$^+$ DCs to up-regulate langerin in vitro and reinforces the idea that CD1c DCs could function as LC precursors during inflammation and potentially give rise to LCH cells. Some of the key differences in gene expression profile between LCH cells and LCs are lost when LCH cells are compared with langerin$^+$ CD1c$^+$ DCs. For example, langerin$^+$ DCs are EpCAM and E-cadherin negative and have higher CD11b and CD11c, unlike LCs.[75] Direct comparison of the transcriptional profiles of LCH with blood CD1c$^+$ DCs and epidermal LCs indicates similar proximity[61] but further studies are required to compare LCH with tissue CD1c$^+$ DCs and langerin$^+$ in vitro–derived CD1c$^+$ DCs in detail.

REVISITING THE CELL OF ORIGIN IN LANGERHANS CELL HISTIOCYTOSIS
Lineage Tracing Langerhans Cell Histiocytosis

Somatic mutations in LCH have provided a foothold with which to study the cell of origin of LCH. As discussed previously, it is evident that LCH cells could arise from more than 1 source. In an attempt to more precisely identify candidate precursor populations, the authors asked whether the mutation encoding BRAF V600E was present in circulating mononuclear cells in patients with active LCH. In the authors' series of 100 patients, peripheral blood mononuclear cells with the BRAF V600E point mutation were identified in all patients with high-risk LCH in whom BRAF V600E was detected in lesion LCH cells.[77] No circulating cells with BRAF V600E were identified in patients with single-system disease and only in a small number of patients with presumed multifocal low-risk disease. Furthermore, the presence of circulating cells in high-risk patients correlated with disease activity. Lineage analysis of the circulating cells in high-risk patients identified cells with BRAF V600E in CD14$^+$ monocyte and CD11c$^+$ myeloid DCs (which includes CD1c$^+$ DCs, CD141$^+$ DCs, and CD16$^+$ nonclassical monocytes) fractions in all cases, suggesting the somatic mutation arose in a myeloid progenitor.

Continuing the search upstream for the hematopoietic origin of LCH, analysis of bone marrow aspirate demonstrated that the BRAF V600E mutation was present in CD34$^+$ hematopoietic stem and progenitor cells (HSPCs) in some, but not all, cases of high-risk patients. In half of the cases where BRAF V600E was identified in bone marrow aspirate, histology was reportedly normal, suggesting the mutation arose in morphologically normal precursor cells. In cases of BRAF V600E identified in CD34$^+$ HSPCs, it could also be identified in circulating CD19$^+$ B cells, suggesting the involvement of a pluripotent stem cells. CD3$^+$ T cells were not affected in keeping with their relative independence from the bone marrow.[77] BRAF V600E was also recently identified in CD34$^+$ cells of patients with hairy cell leukemia.[78] It is not clear why the same presumed driver mutation occurring in hematopoietic stem cells leads to distinct conditions. Potential explanations include epigenetic imprinting of individual stem cells toward different fates or additional modifying somatic mutations[79] or acquisition of mutations at different stages of hematopoietic development.

An Updated Model of Langerhans Cell Histiocytosis

These data suggest a revised model of LCH pathogenesis in which the developmental stage at which an ERK-activating mutation arises determines the clinical manifestations (see **Fig. 2B**). The common histology observed by Lichtenstein[80] could represent a common final pathway from many different starting points. This hypothesis is further supported by the observation that enforced expression of BRAF V600E in langerin$^+$ cells in mice resulted in formation of localized LCH-like lesions, with no BRAF V600E expressed in cells in circulation, whereas enforced expression of BRAF V600E in CD11c$^+$ cells resulted in a more aggressive phenotype similar to disseminated high-risk LCH.[77]

Juvenile Xanthogranuloma and Erdheim-Chester Disease: Cousins or Siblings of Langerhans Cell Histiocytosis?

Juvenile xanthogranuloma (JXG) and Erdheim-Chester disease (ECD) are histologically similar diseases characterized by CD14$^+$, CD68$^+$, fascin$^+$, factor XIII$^+$, CD1a$^+$, and CD207$^-$ histiocytes. JXG is a disease of childhood that, like LCH, ranges from trivial skin-limited lesions to life-threatening disseminated disease. JXG has been reported to copresent with juvenile myelomonocytic leukemia as well as with germline mutations in *NF1* that implicate potential role for MAPK hyperactivity in pathogenesis (reviewed by Berres and colleagues[81]). ECD is a rare disease of adults that typically presents with more clinically ominous systemic lesions. Like LCH, BRAF V600E and other activating MAPK mutations are reported in a majority of cases.[82,83] Furthermore, both JXG and ECD have been reported to copresent with LCH, either with mixed histology in the same lesion or with distinct histology in different lesions (reviewed by Berres and colleagues[81]). Together, the common trigger of MAPK hyperactivity and consistent mutations across lesions in patients with mixed histiocytic disorders[29,77,84] suggest potential for a common origin and blurs the distinction between the neoplastic histiocytoses.

Langerhans Cell Histiocytosis as a Myeloproliferative Disorder

Activating somatic mutations in hematopoietic stem cells and myeloid precursors in LCH patients, coupled with the formation of lesions driven by BRAF V600E in mouse models, support the classification of LCH as a myeloid neoplasia. Transformed DC clones presumably recruit inflammatory cells, resulting in a cytokine rich milieu that promotes LCH cell survival. The authors, therefore, propose that LCH and related JXG and ECD represent a class of histiocytic inflammatory myeloproliferative neoplastic disorder. Other myeloproliferative neoplastic disorders, such as chronic myelogenous leukemia and myelofibrosis, share the features of a genetically quiet landscape with single-driver mutations in kinase pathways and a prominent inflammatory component to disease.

Rebranding LCH as a bona fide myeloid neoplasia has some practical as well as political implications. First, understanding LCH as a stem cell disease may explain the high rate of relapse in patients treated with local or minimally myelotoxic therapeutic strategies.[85] If approached as a stem cell disease, optimal therapy for patients with systemic disease would focus on eradicating the transformed precursor rather than treating individual lesions or tolerating frequent reactivations. Furthermore, chemotherapy agents with efficacy against myleloid lineages may have superior efficacy in LCH compared with traditional acute lymphocytic leukemia–based therapies. In keeping with this, small cohort studies report that clofarabine, a nucleoside analogue with efficacy in acute myeloid leukemia, has cured some patients with aggressive, refractory LCH.[86–88] Finally, direct targeted therapy with RAF inhibitors, such as vemurafenib, has shown early promise in adults with ECD and LCH, further demonstrating the critical role of MAPK activation in driving pathogenesis.[89]

SUMMARY/FUTURE DIRECTIONS

LCH is a complex disease with a fascinating history. Individual reports of highly variable intriguing presentations merged into eponymous classifications that were later unified as histiocytosis X, due to common histology. Subsequently, LCH shifted focus to the aberrant development of LCs. New data support a model that once again deconstructs this single diagnosis into its many facets, each caused by a repertoire of mutations acting at multiple stages of myeloid cell development. The common molecular pathway is MAPK hyperactivation and the common endpoint is a $CD1a^+$ $CD1c^+$ neoplastic cell, but it now seems that every patient has a own private route to developing LCH.

The pace of progress since the last LCH edition of *Hematology/Oncology Clinics of North America* has accelerated, although patients continue to have suboptimal outcomes, and many fundamental aspects of pathogenesis remain unanswered. Politically, new understanding of the nature of LCH is highly significant in placing LCH in the disease family embraced by funding agencies, including the National Cancer Institute, as well as by cooperative clinical trial and translational research groups that advocate for patients with cancer and related disorders. Scientifically, the mechanisms by which MAPK activation drives differentiation of the precursor and subsequent recruitment of inflammatory infiltrate are not known. Improved understanding of mechanisms of pathogenesis will further inform general clinical approaches as well as opportunities for personalized approaches to risk stratification, targeted therapy, and monitoring disease burden. Although much remains to be learned, the authors believe that there is now a more rational path to develop strategy to improve outcomes for patients with LCH beyond the luck of the roulette wheel.

REFERENCES

1. Van Furth R, Cohn ZA. The origin and kinetics of mononuclear phagocytes. J Exp Med 1968;128:415–35.
2. Guilliams M, Ginhoux F, Jakubzick C, et al. Dendritic cells, monocytes and macrophages: a unified nomenclature based on ontogeny. Nat Rev Immunol 2014;14: 571–8.
3. Geissmann F, Manz MG, Jung S, et al. Development of monocytes, macrophages, and dendritic cells. Science 2010;327:656–61.
4. Collin M, McGovern N, Haniffa M. Human dendritic cell subsets. Immunology 2013;140:22–30.
5. Nezelof C, Basset F, Rousseau MF. Histiocytosis X histogenetic arguments for a Langerhans cell origin. Biomedicine 1973;18:365–71.
6. Arceci RJ, Brenner MK, Pritchard J. Controversies and new approaches to treatment of Langerhans cell histiocytosis. Hematol Oncol Clin North Am 1998;12: 339–57.
7. Gadner H, Grois N, Arico M, et al. A randomized trial of treatment for multisystem Langerhans' cell histiocytosis. J Pediatr 2001;138:728–34.
8. Gadner H, Grois N, Potschger U, et al. Improved outcome in multisystem Langerhans cell histiocytosis is associated with therapy intensification. Blood 2008; 111:2556–62.
9. Degar BA, Rollins BJ. Langerhans cell histiocytosis: malignancy or inflammatory disorder doing a great job of imitating one? Dis Model Mech 2009;2:436–9.
10. Jeziorski E, Senechal B, Molina TJ, et al. Herpes-virus infection in patients with Langerhans cell histiocytosis: a case-controlled sero-epidemiological study, and in situ analysis. PLoS One 2008;3:e3262.

11. Nezelof C, Basset F. An hypothesis Langerhans cell histiocytosis: the failure of the immune system to switch from an innate to an adaptive mode. Pediatr Blood Cancer 2004;42:398–400.
12. Geissmann F, Lepelletier Y, Fraitag S, et al. Differentiation of Langerhans cells in Langerhans cell histiocytosis. Blood 2001;97:1241–8.
13. Fleming MD, Pinkus JL, Fournier MV, et al. Coincident expression of the chemokine receptors CCR6 and CCR7 by pathologic Langerhans cells in Langerhans cell histiocytosis. Blood 2003;101:2473–5.
14. Annels NE, da Costa CE, Prins FA, et al. Aberrant chemokine receptor expression and chemokine production by Langerhans cells underlies the pathogenesis of Langerhans cell histiocytosis. J Exp Med 2003;197:1385–90.
15. Laman JD, Leenen PJ, Annels NE, et al. Langerhans-cell histiocytosis 'insight into DC biology'. Trends Immunol 2003;24:190–6.
16. Egeler RM, Neglia JP, Arico M, et al. The relation of Langerhans cell histiocytosis to acute leukemia, lymphomas, and other solid tumors. The LCH-Malignancy Study Group of the Histiocyte Society. Hematol Oncol Clin North Am 1998;12: 369–78.
17. Surico G, Muggeo P, Rigillo N, et al. Concurrent Langerhans cell histiocytosis and myelodysplasia in children. Med Pediatr Oncol 2000;35:421–5.
18. Willman CL, Busque L, Griffith BB, et al. Langerhans'-cell histiocytosis (histiocytosis X)–a clonal proliferative disease. N Engl J Med 1994;331:154–60.
19. Yu RC, Chu C, Buluwela L, et al. Clonal proliferation of Langerhans cells in Langerhans cell histiocytosis. Lancet 1994;343:767–8.
20. Waskow C, Liu K, Darrasse-Jeze G, et al. The receptor tyrosine kinase Flt3 is required for dendritic cell development in peripheral lymphoid tissues. Nat Immunol 2008;9:676–83.
21. Senechal B, Elain G, Jeziorski E, et al. Expansion of regulatory T cells in patients with Langerhans cell histiocytosis. PLoS Med 2007;4:e253.
22. Merad M, Manz MG, Karsunky H, et al. Langerhans cells renew in the skin throughout life under steady-state conditions. Nat Immunol 2002;3:1135–41.
23. da Costa CE, Szuhai K, van ER, et al. No genomic aberrations in Langerhans cell histiocytosis as assessed by diverse molecular technologies. Genes Chromosomes Cancer 2009;48:239–49.
24. Badalian-Very G, Vergilio JA, Degar BA, et al. Recurrent BRAF mutations in Langerhans cell histiocytosis. Blood 2010;116:1919–23.
25. Maurer G, Tarkowski B, Baccarini M. Raf kinases in cancer-roles and therapeutic opportunities. Oncogene 2011;30:3477–88.
26. Michaloglou C, Vredeveld LC, Mooi WJ, et al. BRAF(E600) in benign and malignant human tumours. Oncogene 2008;27:877–95.
27. Davies H, Bignell GR, Cox C, et al. Mutations of the BRAF gene in human cancer. Nature 2002;417:949–54.
28. Nelson DS, Quispel W, Badalian-Very G, et al. Somatic activating ARAF mutations in Langerhans cell histiocytosis. Blood 2014;123:3152–5.
29. Chakraborty R, Hampton OA, Shen X, et al. Mutually exclusive recurrent somatic mutations in MAP2K1 and BRAF support a central role for ERK activation in LCH pathogenesis. Blood 2014;124:3007–15.
30. Brown NA, Furtado LV, Betz BL, et al. High prevalence of somatic MAP2K1 mutations in BRAF V600E-negative Langerhans cell histiocytosis. Blood 2014; 124:1655–8.
31. Rollin BJ. Genomic alterations in langerhans cell histiocytosis. Journal of Hematology & Oncology 2015, in press.

32. Nezelof C, Basset F. From histiocytosis X to Langerhans cell histiocytosis: a personal account. Int J Surg Pathol 2001;9:137–46.

33. Breathnach AS, Gross M, Basset F, et al. Freeze-fracture replication of X-granules in cells of cutaneous lesions of histiocytosis-X. Br J Dermatol 1973;89. p. 571–85.

34. Valladeau J, Ravel O, Dezutter-Dambuyant C, et al. Langerin, a novel C-type lectin specific to Langerhans cells, is an endocytic receptor that induces the formation of Birbeck granules. Immunity 2000;12:71–81.

35. Chikwava K, Jaffe R. Langerin (CD207) staining in normal pediatric tissues, reactive lymph nodes, and childhood histiocytic disorders. Pediatr Dev Pathol 2004;7: 607–14.

36. Peters TL, McClain KL, Allen CE. Neither IL-17A mRNA nor IL-17A protein are detectable in Langerhans cell histiocytosis lesions. Mol Ther 2011;19:1433–9.

37. Coury F, Annels N, Rivollier A, et al. Langerhans cell histiocytosis reveals a new IL-17A-dependent pathway of dendritic cell fusion. Nat Med 2008;14:81–7.

38. Sahm F, Capper D, Preusser M, et al. BRAFV600E mutant protein is expressed in cells of variable maturation in Langerhans cell histiocytosis. Blood 2012;120: e28–34.

39. Allen CE, Li L, Peters TL, et al. Cell-specific gene expression in Langerhans cell histiocytosis lesions reveals a distinct profile compared with epidermal Langerhans cells. J Immunol 2010;184:4557–67.

40. Romani N, Clausen BE, Stoitzner P. Langerhans cells and more: langerin-expressing dendritic cell subsets in the skin. Immunol Rev 2010;234:120–41.

41. Schuster C, Vaculik C, Fiala C, et al. HLA-DR+ leukocytes acquire CD1 antigens in embryonic and fetal human skin and contain functional antigen-presenting cells. J Exp Med 2009;206:169–81.

42. Hoeffel G, Wang Y, Greter M, et al. Adult Langerhans cells derive predominantly from embryonic fetal liver monocytes with a minor contribution of yolk sac-derived macrophages. J Exp Med 2012;209:1167–81.

43. Wang Y, Szretter KJ, Vermi W, et al. IL-34 is a tissue-restricted ligand of CSF1R required for the development of Langerhans cells and microglia. Nat Immunol 2012;13:753–60.

44. Greter M, Lelios I, Pelczar P, et al. Stroma-derived interleukin-34 controls the development and maintenance of langerhans cells and the maintenance of microglia. Immunity 2012;37:1050–60.

45. Borkowski TA, Letterio JJ, Farr AG, et al. A role for endogenous transforming growth factor beta 1 in Langerhans cell biology: the skin of transforming growth factor beta 1 null mice is devoid of epidermal Langerhans cells. J Exp Med 1996; 184:2417–22.

46. Schulz C, Gomez PE, Chorro L, et al. A lineage of myeloid cells independent of Myb and hematopoietic stem cells. Science 2012;336:86–90.

47. Boiers C, Carrelha J, Lutteropp M, et al. Lymphomyeloid contribution of an immune-restricted progenitor emerging prior to definitive hematopoietic stem cells. Cell Stem Cell 2013;13:535–48.

48. Gomez PE, Klapproth K, Schulz C, et al. Tissue-resident macrophages originate from yolk-sac-derived erythro-myeloid progenitors. Nature 2015;518:547–51.

49. Czernielewski JM, Demarchez M. Further evidence for the self-reproducing capacity of Langerhans cells in human skin. J Invest Dermatol 1987;88:17–20.

50. Hambleton S, Salem S, Bustamante J, et al. IRF8 mutations and human dendritic-cell immunodeficiency. N Engl J Med 2011;365:127–38.

51. Bigley V, Haniffa M, Doulatov S, et al. The human syndrome of dendritic cell, monocyte, B and NK lymphoid deficiency. J Exp Med 2011;208:227–34.

52. Kanitakis J. Transmission of rosacea from the graft in facial allotransplantation. Am J Transplant 2011;11:1338–9.
53. Collin MP, Hart DN, Jackson GH, et al. The fate of human Langerhans cells in hematopoietic stem cell transplantation. J Exp Med 2006;203:27–33.
54. Mielcarek M, Kirkorian AY, Hackman RC, et al. Langerhans cell homeostasis and turnover after nonmyeloablative and myeloablative allogeneic hematopoietic cell transplantation. Transplantation 2014;98:563–8.
55. Ginhoux F, Tacke F, Angeli V, et al. Langerhans cells arise from monocytes in vivo. Nat Immunol 2006;7:265–73.
56. Sere KM, Lin Q, Felker P, et al. Dendritic cell lineage commitment is instructed by distinct cytokine signals. Eur J Cell Biol 2012;91:515–23.
57. Nagao K, Kobayashi T, Moro K, et al. Stress-induced production of chemokines by hair follicles regulates the trafficking of dendritic cells in skin. Nat Immunol 2012;13:744–52.
58. Kaplan G, Nusrat A, Witmer MD, et al. Distribution and turnover of Langerhans cells during delayed immune responses in human skin. J Exp Med 1987;165:763–76.
59. Geissmann F, Prost C, Monnet JP, et al. Transforming growth factor beta1, in the presence of granulocyte/macrophage colony-stimulating factor and interleukin 4, induces differentiation of human peripheral blood monocytes into dendritic Langerhans cells. J Exp Med 1998;187:961–6.
60. Hoshino N, Katayama N, Shibasaki T, et al. A novel role for Notch ligand Delta-1 as a regulator of human Langerhans cell development from blood monocytes. J Leukoc Biol 2005;78:921–9.
61. Hutter C, Kauer M, Simonitsch-Klupp I, et al. Notch is active in Langerhans cell histiocytosis and confers pathognomonic features on dendritic cells. Blood 2012;120:5199–208.
62. Schaerli P, Willimann K, Ebert LM, et al. Cutaneous CXCL14 targets blood precursors to epidermal niches for Langerhans cell differentiation. Immunity 2005;23: 331–42.
63. McGovern N, Schlitzer A, Gunawan M, et al. Human dermal CD14(+) cells are a transient population of monocyte-derived macrophages. Immunity 2014;41:465–77.
64. Larregina AT, Morelli AE, Spencer LA, et al. Dermal-resident CD14+ cells differentiate into Langerhans cells. Nat Immunol 2001;2:1151–8.
65. Caux C, Vanbervliet B, Massacrier C, et al. CD34+ hematopoietic progenitors from human cord blood differentiate along two independent dendritic cell pathways in response to GM-CSF+TNF alpha. J Exp Med 1996;184: 695–706.
66. Strunk D, Rappersberger K, Egger C, et al. Generation of human dendritic cells/Langerhans cells from circulating CD34+ hematopoietic progenitor cells. Blood 1996;87:1292–302.
67. Martinez-Cingolani C, Grandclaudon M, Jeanmougin M, et al. Human blood BDCA-1 dendritic cells differentiate into Langerhans-like cells with thymic stromal lymphopoietin and TGF-beta. Blood 2014;124:2411–20.
68. Milne P, Bigley V, Gunawan M, et al. CD1c+ blood dendritic cells have Langerhans cell potential. Blood 2015;125:470–3.
69. Jardine L, Barge D, Ames-Draycott A, et al. Rapid detection of dendritic cell and monocyte disorders using CD4 as a lineage marker of the human peripheral blood antigen-presenting cell compartment. Front Immunol 2013;4:495.
70. Haniffa M, Shin A, Bigley V, et al. Human tissues contain CD141hi cross-presenting dendritic cells with functional homology to mouse CD103+ nonlymphoid dendritic cells. Immunity 2012;37:60–73.

71. Yu CI, Becker C, Wang Y, et al. Human CD1c+ dendritic cells drive the differentiation of CD103+ CD8+ mucosal effector T cells via the cytokine TGF-beta. Immunity 2013;38:818–30.

72. Reizis B, Colonna M, Trinchieri G, et al. Plasmacytoid dendritic cells: one-trick ponies or workhorses of the immune system? Nat Rev Immunol 2011;11:558–65.

73. Angel CE, Lala A, Chen CJ, et al. CD14+ antigen-presenting cells in human dermis are less mature than their CD1a+ counterparts. Int Immunol 2007;19: 1271–9.

74. Chu CC, Ali N, Karagiannis P, et al. Resident CD141 (BDCA3)+ dendritic cells in human skin produce IL-10 and induce regulatory T cells that suppress skin inflammation. J Exp Med 2012;209:935–45.

75. Bigley V, McGovern N, Milne P, et al. Langerin-expressing dendritic cells in human tissues are related to CD1c+ dendritic cells and distinct from Langerhans cells and CD141high XCR1+ dendritic cells. J Leukoc Biol 2014;97(4):627–34.

76. Merad M, Ginhoux F, Collin M. Origin, homeostasis and function of Langerhans cells and other langerin-expressing dendritic cells. Nat Rev Immunol 2008;8: 935–47.

77. Berres ML, Lim KP, Peters T, et al. BRAF-V600E expression in precursor versus differentiated dendritic cells defines clinically distinct LCH risk groups. J Exp Med 2014;211:669–83.

78. Chung SS, Kim E, Park JH, et al. Hematopoietic stem cell origin of BRAFV600E mutations in hairy cell leukemia. Sci Transl Med 2014;6:238ra71.

79. Naik SH, Perie L, Swart E, et al. Diverse and heritable lineage imprinting of early haematopoietic progenitors. Nature 2013;496:229–32.

80. Berres ML, Allen CE, Merad M. Pathological consequence of misguided dendritic cell differentiation in histiocytic diseases. Adv Immunol 2013;120:127–61.

81. Lichtenstein L. Histiocytosis X; integration of eosinophilic granuloma of bone, Letterer-Siwe disease, and Schuller-Christian disease as related manifestations of a single nosologic entity. AMA Arch Pathol 1953;56:84–102.

82. Haroche J, Charlotte F, Arnaud L, et al. High prevalence of BRAF V600E mutations in Erdheim-Chester disease but not in other non-Langerhans cell histiocytoses. Blood 2012;120:2700–3.

83. Emile JF, Diamond EL, Helias-Rodzewicz Z, et al. Recurrent RAS and PIK3CA mutations in Erdheim-Chester disease. Blood 2014;124:3016–9.

84. Hervier B, Haroche J, Arnaud L, et al. Association of both Langerhans cell histiocytosis and Erdheim-Chester disease linked to the BRAFV600E mutation. Blood 2014;124:1119–26.

85. Minkov M, Steiner M, Potschger U, et al. Reactivations in multisystem Langerhans cell histiocytosis: data of the international LCH registry. J Pediatr 2008;153:700–5, 705.e1–2.

86. Simko SJ, Tran HD, Jones J, et al. Clofarabine salvage therapy in refractory multifocal histiocytic disorders, including Langerhans cell histiocytosis, juvenile xanthogranuloma and Rosai-Dorfman disease. Pediatr Blood Cancer 2014;61: 479–87.

87. Rodriguez-Galindo C, Jeng M, Khuu P, et al. Clofarabine in refractory Langerhans cell histiocytosis. Pediatr Blood Cancer 2008;51:703–6.

88. Abraham A, Alsultan A, Jeng M, et al. Clofarabine salvage therapy for refractory high-risk langerhans cell histiocytosis. Pediatr Blood Cancer 2013;60:E19–22.

89. Haroche J, Cohen-Aubart F, Emile JF, et al. Dramatic efficacy of vemurafenib in both multisystemic and refractory Erdheim-Chester disease and Langerhans cell histiocytosis harboring the BRAF V600E mutation. Blood 2013;121:1495–500.

Genomic Alterations in Langerhans Cell Histiocytosis

Barrett J. Rollins, MD, PhD[a,b,*]

KEYWORDS

- Langerhans cell histiocytosis • LCH • BRAF • MAP2K1 • MEK1

KEY POINTS

- Recurrent somatic genomic abnormalities occur in Langerhans cell histiocytosis (LCH), indicating that it is a neoplastic disease.
- Most mutations activate signaling enzymes that result in extracellular-signal-regulated kinase (ERK) activation.
- More than 50% of cases carry *BRAF* mutations and 10% to 28% carry *MAP2K1* mutations, but all cases show activation of ERK.
- Significant clinical responses to RAF family inhibitors have been reported in patients whose LCH cells carry *BRAF* mutations, indicating that these mutations are authentic drivers of disease in LCH.

INTRODUCTION

Long considered an enigmatic disease, LCH defies simple categorization. Its 4 clinically distinct syndromes (Hand-Schüller-Christian disease, Letterer-Siwe disease, eosinophilic granuloma, and Hashimoto-Pritzker disease) were unified by observations in the mid-twentieth century of a characteristically abnormal histiocyte with distinctive morphology, subcellular structures, and staining patterns that appears in all forms of the disease.[1–3] Although this categorization has helped clarify thinking about LCH, it has not explained its pathogenesis or its impressively protean clinical manifestations.

The author has no commercial or financial conflicts of interest to declare. The author's work has been supported by the Histiocytosis Association, Team Ippolitte/Deloitte of the Boston Marathon Jimmy Fund Walk, Stichting 1000 Kaarsjes voor Juultje, the Say Yes to Education Foundation, and Mr George Weiss.
^a Department of Medical Oncology, Dana-Farber Cancer Institute, Harvard Medical School, 450 Brookline Avenue, Boston, MA 02215, USA; ^b Department of Medicine, Brigham and Women's Hospital, Harvard Medical School, Boston, MA 02115, USA
* Department of Medical Oncology, Dana-Farber Cancer Institute, 450 Brookline Avenue, Boston, MA 02215.
E-mail address: barrett_rollins@dfci.harvard.edu

Hematol Oncol Clin N Am 29 (2015) 839–851
http://dx.doi.org/10.1016/j.hoc.2015.06.004
0889-8588/15/$ – see front matter © 2015 Elsevier Inc. All rights reserved.

Further progress in characterizing LCH has been impeded by a paucity of samples, a consequence both of the low prevalence of LCH[4,5] and the small size of most tissue samples obtained for clinical purposes. However, technical advances in the genomic analysis of clinical material have been applied to LCH and have revolutionized the understanding of the fundamental nature of the disease. One of the most enabling innovations is the ability to perform robust multiplexed genetic testing on small amounts of archived clinical material, that is, formalin-fixed, paraffin-embedded samples acquired for diagnostic purposes.[6–8] This ability has opened the archives of pathology departments around the world to genomic analyses, and the application of these technologies has revealed some of the first evidence for recurrent and pathogenetically relevant mutations in LCH. To date, these have been somatic mutations rather than germline alterations affecting risk. The result has been a clearer understanding of LCH as a neoplastic disease and the identification of therapeutically important molecular targets.

MITOGEN-ACTIVATED PROTEIN KINASE PATHWAY ACTIVATION
BRAF

One of the first technologies capable of testing archived human samples for multiple alleles simultaneously was the Sequenom mass spectrometric genotyping platform.[6] A modification specific for oncology applications known as OncoMap, which tests 983 specific mutations in 115 cancer-related genes, was applied to 61 LCH clinical samples.[9] Overall, very few mutations were detected, a common finding in all subsequent studies (see later discussion) attesting to the stability of the LCH genome. However, a mutation in BRAF encoding the substitution of glutamate for valine at amino acid 600 (BRAF V600E) was observed in 57% of the samples.[9] This mutation, which produces a constitutively active BRAF kinase, is the most commonly observed BRAF variant in cancer and is found in a variety of different cancer types in which it often plays a driver role in pathogenesis.[10–14] The effect of mutationally activated BRAF is to stimulate signaling through the RAS/RAF/MEK/ERK pathway leading to constitutive transcription of genes involved in a variety of cellular responses including proliferation (**Fig. 1**).

The presence in LCH of recurrent activating mutations in BRAF has been confirmed in several studies using a variety of different detection techniques (**Table 1**). Among them are immunohistochemical studies with a V600E-specific antibody, which confirms that the variant is present specifically in LCH histiocytes,[15] a fact that could previously be inferred only indirectly by molecular means.[9] BRAF mutations occur in all clinical settings, including pediatric, adult, single system, and multisystem disease, and their overall prevalence in reported studies is 45% to 65%.[9,15–24] Surprisingly, BRAF mutations appear at a nearly similar frequency in pulmonary LCH, a disease of adult smokers that has generally been thought to be polyclonal. However, about one-third of pulmonary LCH cases are clonal.[25] It is also possible that cases that are polyclonal in the aggregate actually comprise several clones of BRAF mutant disease that arose independently.

In the original OncoMap analysis, the median age of patients whose histiocytes contain BRAF V600E was less than the median age of patients whose histiocytes did not, and younger age was associated with the presence of the mutation in an unadjusted exact logistic model but not in the adjusted model.[9] The presence of mutated BRAF did not correlate with any other clinical features, although the clinical annotation of that sample set was limited. In contrast, in the largest sample set analyzed to date, clinical annotation was much more complete and the presence of BRAF V600E

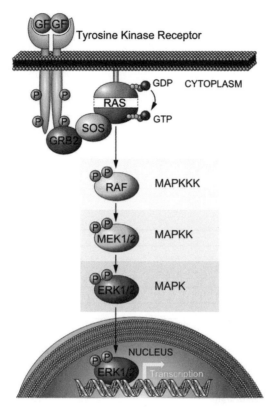

Fig. 1. The ERK signal transduction cascade. The ERK signaling cascade transmits stimuli for a variety of cellular responses, such as proliferation, from the cell surface to the nucleus. In this example, engagement of a tyrosine kinase growth factor receptor by its cognate ligand leads to phosphorylation of amino acids in the cytoplasmic domain of the receptor, which, in turn, activates RAS through GRB2 and SOS. Activated RAS activates RAF through phosphorylation; activated RAF phosphorylates and activates MEK1/2; activated MEK1/2 phosphorylates ERK1/2, which then translocates to the nucleus to stimulate transcription of genes involved in cell proliferation. RAF, MEK1/2, and ERK1/2 are members of the mitogen-activated protein (MAP) kinase kinase kinase (MAPKKK), MAP kinase kinase (MAPKK), and MAP kinase (MAPK) families, respectively (see **Fig. 2**). Constitutive activation of components of this cascade would produce constitutive transcription of target genes and unrestrained cell proliferation. This class of activating mutations in genes encoding RAF proteins (BRAF and ARAF) and MEK1 has been described in LCH (see text).

correlated with disease relapse.[16] That study also identified BRAF V600E in bone marrow–derived hematopoietic precursors from patients with high-risk LCH. In patients with low-risk disease, the mutation was detected only in lesional cells. This finding suggests that the appearance of a driver mutation earlier in ontogeny might lead to a more widely disseminated and aggressive form of LCH.

Like other BRAF-driven diseases, LCH is also associated with activating mutations of *BRAF* other than V600E. For example, another acidic amino acid substitution for V600, BRAF V600D (a substitution of aspartate for valine), is an activating mutation that occurs rarely in melanoma[10] and has been reported in a single case of LCH.[26] A more commonly observed *BRAF* variant in melanoma, BRAF V600K (a substitution

Table 1
Prevalence of *BRAF* mutations in LCH

Report	Prevalence[a] (%)
Badalian-Very et al,[9] 2010	57 (35/61)
	42 (5/12) pulmonary only
	61 (30/49) extrapulmonary
Haroche et al,[19] 2012	38 (11/29)
Sahm et al,[15] 2012	38 (34/89)[b,c]
Satoh et al,[22] 2012	56 (9/16)[c]
Wei et al,[24] 2013	56 (28/50)
	100 (1/1) pulmonary only
	55 (27/49) extrapulmonary
Roden et al,[21] 2014	33 (26/79)
	28 (7/25) pulmonary only
	35 (19/54) extrapulmonary
Berres et al,[16] 2014	64 (64/100)[c]
Chilosi et al,[18] 2014	46 (18/38)
	63 (12/19) pulmonary only
	32 (6/19) extrapulmonary
Méhes et al,[20] 2014	53 (8/15)
Varga et al,[23] 2014	54 (6/11) adult cutaneous
Bubolz et al,[17] 2014	48 (23/48)
	25 (1/4) pulmonary only
	50 (22/44) extrapulmonary

The prevalence of any mutation in *BRAF* was taken from the indicated reference. When disease involving only the lungs (pulmonary only) was described, the prevalence of *BRAF* mutations in that disease subtype is indicated.

[a] Prevalence is indicated with actual numbers shown in parentheses (number of cases with mutated *BRAF*/total number of cases).
[b] Detected by immunohistochemistry using VE-1 antibody.
[c] No pulmonary only cases.
Data from Refs.[9,15–24]

of lysine for valine),[27] has not yet been reported in LCH. In addition, an insertional mutation substituting an additional 4 amino acids, DLAT (aspartate-leucine-alanine-threonine), for valine at amino acid position 600 has been found in a single LCH case.[22] Although this variant has not been tested directly for constitutive kinase activity, structural inferences suggest that its effects on constitutive activation of BRAF kinase should be similar to that of V600E.

ARAF

Although activating BRAF mutations are present in 45% to 65% of LCH cases, the histiocytes in all LCH cases examined to date show high levels of phosphorylated ERK, implying ERK pathway activation[9,16] (see **Fig. 1**). This finding has led several groups to perform even broader analyses such as whole-exome sequencing to find mechanisms for ERK activation other than activating *BRAF* mutations.[16,28] A surprising outcome of one whole-exome analysis was the discovery of an activating mutation of *ARAF*.[28] ARAF is another mitogen-activated protein (MAP) kinase kinase kinase in the same protein family as BRAF (**Fig. 2**). The *ARAF* abnormality discovered in this study was actually a compound mutation comprising a single base substitution encoding leucine in place of phenylalanine at position 351 (F351L) and a 6-nucleotide deletion leading to

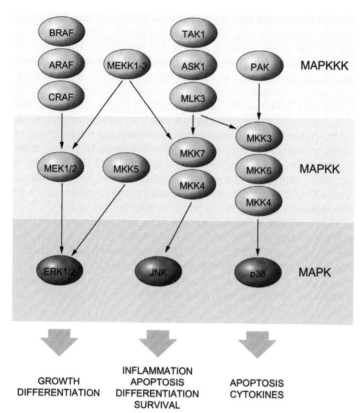

Fig. 2. MAP kinase families. Signaling from the cell surface to the nucleus occurs through serial activation of members of the MAP kinase family of proteins. Generically, signaling proceeds from MAP kinase kinase kinase (MAPKKK) enzymes to MAP kinase kinase (MAPKK) enzymes and then to MAP kinase (MAPK) enzymes. **Fig. 1** described the specific enzymes involved in growth and differentiation, portrayed here as the leftmost cascade. Other cascades result in activation of the MAP kinase JNK, which influences inflammation, apoptosis, differentiation, and survival, and the MAP kinase p38, which influences apoptosis and the release of cytokines. Note that there is cross talk between these cascades. In particular, the MAPKKKs MEKK1–3 stimulate the JNK pathway but can also stimulate the ERK1/2 pathway.

loss of amino acids 347 and 348 (Q347_A348del). Biochemical analysis of this variant demonstrated that it is a constitutively active kinase capable of transforming mouse embryo fibroblasts, suggesting that it is likely to be a driver mutation in this clinical case. This ARAF variant was sensitive to inhibition by vemurafenib in vitro.

A distinct *ARAF* mutation, T70M (methionine substituted for threonine at position 70), has also been described in a single mixed case of LCH and Erdheim-Chester disease (ECD).[29] Although this variant, which appears in the COSMIC (Catalog of Somatic Mutations in Cancer) database, has not been tested for RAF kinase activity, it is unlikely to be activated because it appeared in a case that also carried a BRAF V600E mutation. To date, no mutations in *CRAF* (also known as RAF1) have been described in LCH.

MAP2K1

Ongoing sequence analysis of LCH samples has uncovered additional somatic mutations that activate the ERK pathway. Most prominent are activating mutations in

MAP2K1, which encodes the MAP kinase kinase MEK1 (see **Fig. 2**). These mutations are found only in cases carrying wild-type *BRAF* alleles, supporting the notion that they are acting in the same signaling pathway as BRAF.[29–31] The true prevalence of *MAP2K1* mutations is uncertain at present because their frequency differs substantially among the samples tested in various reports: 28% in a 40-sample cohort,[30] 19% in a different 36-sample cohort (of a 41-sample collection that included some mixed LCH/ECD and LCH/juvenile xanthogranuloma cases),[29] and 10% in a 30 sample cohort.[31] It is possible that this disparity arises from differences in the clinical characteristics of the patients who comprised these cohorts, but the presence of *MAP2K1* mutations does not correlate with age, sex, sites of disease, or stage in these studies.

MAP2K1 mutations in LCH cluster vary specifically in 2 domains: an N-terminal negative regulatory domain and the N-terminal portion of the core kinase domain (**Table 2**). Some *MAP2K1* mutations found in solid tumors, leukemias, or lymphomas overlap these regions, but many more occur throughout the protein.[32–36] Among the mutations in LCH are several that result in the same alterations of the MAP2K1 protein but involve different nucleotide substitutions (see **Table 2**). For example, the substitution of serine for cysteine at position 121 (C121S) is created both by a substitution of G for C at nucleotide position 362, an alteration also observed in melanoma,[35] and by a substitution of A for T at position 361, creating a differently mutated codon that nonetheless still encodes serine at amino acid 121. Similarly, the deletion of amino acids

Table 2
MAP2K1 mutations in LCH

Nucleotide Position (Number of Samples)	Amino Acid Position
Negative Regulatory Domain	
140G>A[30](1)	R47Q
159_173del[29,30](2)	F53_Q58delinsL
166_181del>C[31](1)	F56_G61delinsR
167A>C[29](1)	Q56P
168_182del[30](1)	K57_G61del
170_184del[29](1)	Q58_E62del
172_186del[29](2)	Q58_E62del
Kinase Domain	
361T>A/383G>T[30](1)	C121S/G128V
361T>A[31](1)	C121S
362G>C/383G>A[31](1)	C121S/G128D
302_307del[29](1)	E102_I103del
303_308del[30](2)	E102_I103del
304_309del[30](2)	E102_I103del
299_307delinsCTC[30](1)	H100_I103delinsPL
295_312del[30](1)	I99_K104del
Both	
145C>T/316G>A[30](1)	R49C/A106T

Mutations in *MAP2K1* were taken from the published literature. The table sorts them into mutations that occur in the negative regulatory domain and the kinase domain. One case had mutations in both domains. The number of reported cases with the indicated mutation is shown in parentheses.
Data from Refs.[29–31]

58 through 62 arises through an in-frame deletion of nucleotides 303 through 308 or 304 through 309. Finally, the frequently observed deletion of glutamate at position 102 (E102) and isoleucine at position 103 (I103) is produced through in-frame deletions starting at nucleotides 302, 303, or 304. This finding almost certainly reflects substantial selective pressure for these particular variant proteins, which can arise through a variety of alterations at the DNA level, which may be context- or patient specific.

These 2 regions of frequent mutation in LCH cases overlap those reported in variant hairy-cell leukemia or IGHV-34-positive classic hairy-cell leukemia, which, unlike nearly all true classic hairy-cell leukemia, do not carry *BRAF* mutations.[34] The frequency of *MAP2K1* mutations in these wild-type *BRAF* variants is 48%, close to the frequency in wild-type *BRAF* cases reported in one of the LCH cohorts.[30]

Several of these variants have been tested biochemically and found to have constitutive MEK kinase activity.[29,31] Some of the deletion variants have not been tested directly but are presumed also to be constitutive MEK kinases because the deleted regions overlap those that occur in variants known to be constitutively active. In at least 1 case, C121S/G128D, the effect of 2 simultaneous mutations in a single allele has been examined.[31] The single C121S variant has considerable MEK kinase activity in vitro. The G128D substitution (aspartate for glycine at position 121), which has not been described as occurring by itself in LCH or any other disease, leads to some constitutive MEK kinase activity but far less than that of C121S. However, the variant carrying both substitutions is a more active kinase than C121S. This synergistic effect of 2 mutations is reminiscent of the *ARAF* mutations described earlier in which the presence of F351L, which is a weak kinase by itself, greatly enhances the ERK kinase activity of the Q347_A348del deletion.[28]

MAP3K1

In the course of performing whole-exome sequencing on LCH samples, 2 mutations have been discovered in *MAP3K1*, which encodes MEKK1.[28] Both are frameshift deletions leading to truncated proteins: T799fs (a frameshift truncation at threonine at position 799) and L1481fs (a frameshift truncation at leucine at position 1481). (A third variant identified in the same study, E1286V [valine substituted for glutamate at position 1286], was presumed to be a germline single nucleotide polymorphism.) The effects of these mutations on ERK activation are unclear. Although *MAP3K1* encodes the MAP kinase kinase kinase MEKK1 (see **Fig. 2**), which is capable of phosphorylating MEK1,[37] the variants found in LCH were unable to be expressed, including the L1481fs variant in which the truncation is near the protein's C-terminus, suggesting that the variant is unstable. Thus, these are likely to be null alleles as are a large number of MAP3K1 variants in solid tumors such as breast cancers.[38] The mechanisms by which these variants promote neoplastic growth are still unknown but may involve enhanced cell survival through activation of JNK (c-Jun N-terminal kinase) (see **Fig. 2**). In the absence of enhanced MEK1 kinase activity, these variants are unlikely to be contributing directly to ERK activation. This idea is supported by the observation that the T799fs variant occurs in a case that also carries BRAF V600E.

NRAS

A somatic *NRAS* mutation has been described in a case of mixed juvenile myelomonocytic leukemia (JMML) and LCH, the latter based on a CD1a-positive cutaneous infiltrate of characteristic cells.[39] Although this is a genomic abnormality characteristic of JMML, upregulation of the ERK signaling pathway through NRAS activation could also drive LCH. *NRAS* mutations, including Q61R (a substitution of arginine for glutamine at position 61), a known pathogenetic variant, have been described in *BRAF* wild type ECD.[40,41] This finding may be relevant to LCH considering the frequent appearance of LCH/ECD overlap syndromes.

PIK3CA

Because a patient with multisystem LCH experienced a prolonged clinical response to a pan-AKT inhibitor,[42] mutationally activated PIK3CA (phosphatidyl inositol-4,5-bisphosphate 3-kinase, catalytic subunit alpha) was anticipated to be a major driver in this disease. Four hotspot mutational sites in *PIK3CA* (encoding E542K, E545K, A1046T, and H1047R) have been assayed in LCH samples from 86 patients.[43] However, only 1 sample was identified in which a mutation encoding the E542K variant (lysine substituted for glutamate at position 542) was found; this sample did not contain BRAF V600E. This study is limited by its inability to detect any *PIK3CA* mutations other than these 4 hotspots. However, the low frequency of *PIK3CA* mutations in LCH inferred from this work is likely to be accurate because none of the whole-exome sequencing analyses reported to date describe mutations in *PIK3CA*.[28,29]

Tumor Protein 53

Most LCH cases show increased expression of tumor protein p53 (TP53) as determined by immunohistochemistry.[44] Although this suggests the possibility of an abnormality in the TP53 pathway, mutations in TP53 are rare. A single report describes an LCH case containing the R175H variant (histidine substituted for arginine at position 175), which has been characterized as a cancer-associated abnormality.[9,45–47] To date, no mutations in the TP53 regulator MDM2 (mouse double minute 2 homolog) have been described.[28,29,44,48] It is still possible that TP53 overexpression is a driver abnormality in LCH and that it occurs as the result of mechanisms such as epigenetic dysregulation that have not yet been tested in LCH samples. However, its near universality in LCH parallels that of ERK activation and suggests that TP53 overexpression may occur in response to constitutive activation of RAS-RAF-MEK-ERK pathway.

Others

Few additional DNA variants have been described in LCH. In one survey of a small number of LCH cases by whole-exome sequencing, no other potentially relevant substitutions or deletions were described.[28] In another whole-exome sequencing study of 41 cases, 29 mutations targeted the RAS-RAF-MEK-ERK pathway, whereas 23 were nonrecurrent in a variety of genes, including *PICK1* and *PIK3R2*, which, although not directly in that pathway, might theoretically affect ERK activation.[29] Among these was a substitution encoding ERBB3 P921Q (glutamine substituted for proline at position 921), which occurred in a *BRAF* wild type case.

Translocations and Copy Number Changes

Before the era of next-generation sequencing, some analyses suggested the presence of chromosome-level alterations in LCH. One report described a clonal t(7;12)(q11.2;p13) translocation in 1 case as well as nonclonal translocations in this case and 3 more.[49] Since then, however, there have been no additional reports of this or any other translocation in LCH. A careful study of 31 samples found no translocations and documented diploid genomes in all cases.[48]

Copy number changes have been investigated using array comparative genomic hybridization (CGH) and quantitative polymerase chain reaction (PCR). One study applied array CGH to 7 bone lesions and found several copy number alterations scattered through the genome and recurrent loss of heterozygosity at some loci.[50] PCR analysis of a 24-sample set documented fractional allelic loss in LCH samples, which was more frequent in patients with multisystem disease than in those with single-system or low-risk disease.[51] However, these findings were not confirmed in a later study that used high-density single nucleotide polymorphism arrays.[48]

Based on the absence of recurrent chromosomal abnormalities in these reports, it may not be surprising that whole-exome sequencing analyses have also failed to identify recurrent copy number changes or translocations in LCH samples.

CLINICAL IMPLICATIONS

The discovery of activating *BRAF* and *MAP2K1* mutations in LCH suggests the possibility that RAF and MEK1 inhibitors might be clinically useful. To date, however, only scattered case reports support this notion. For example, among 3 patients with BRAF V600E-positive ECD who were treated with the RAF inhibitor vemurafenib, 2 also had LCH involving skin or lymph nodes.[52] Vemurafenib led to striking clinical responses in both the ECD and LCH components in the 2 patients with mixed disease. The response lasted throughout the 4-month period of ongoing treatment and observation. A follow-up study reported on vemurafenib treatment of 8 patients with ECD BRAF V600E-positive ECD, 4 of whom had concurrent LCH.[53] Responses were again seen in all patients, and no resistance was observed during the follow-up period of 6 to 16 months.

In another report, a 45-year-old woman with pure, BRAF V600E-positive LCH who had become refractory to standard treatment (steroids and vinblastine and then cladribine) responded dramatically to vemurafenib.[17] Within 6 weeks of treatment, metabolic activity of her LCH lesions as measured by PET (positron emission tomography) with fludeoxyglucose had returned to background and her anatomic lesions had stabilized. Unfortunately, local regulations required discontinuation of this off-label use of vemurafenib after 12 weeks of treatment. Her disease progressed 6 months later.

Definitive assessment of the efficacy of RAF inhibition in LCH requires trials that attempt to measure this directly. Clinical trials are open at the time of this writing that may fulfill this need, such as a trial of dabrafenib in children and adolescents with BRAF V600 mutation-positive diseases, including LCH (NCT01677741). The presence of *MAP2K1* mutations in *BRAF* wild-type LCH suggests that MEK1 inhibitors such as trametinib need to be tested. By analogy to other diseases such as melanoma, treatment with both a RAF inhibitor and a MEK1 inhibitor, such as trametinib, may prevent the appearance of resistance.[54] Such a trial of trametinib in combination with dabrafenib in children and adolescents with BRAF V600 mutation-positive diseases including LCH has been started (NCT02124772).

SUMMARY

The application of advanced genomic analytical technologies to LCH has led to a new and deeper understanding of this disease. These tools have revealed recurrent mutations in RAF and MEK family members, indicating that LCH is a neoplasm driven by ERK pathway activation. This inference is tentatively supported by the striking clinical responses to RAF inhibitors in patients whose LCH cells carry BRAF V600E mutations, including patients who have failed first- and second-line therapies.[17,52,53] Rigorous demonstration of the pathogenetic role of ERK pathway mutations in LCH awaits completion of trials of RAF and MEK inhibitors.

Mutations in RAF and MEK family members are found in 70% to 75% of LCH cases.[9,15–24] The fact that ERK activation has been documented in all cases examined to date[9,16] means that the causes for this activation remain unknown in 25% to 30% of LCH cases. Although the total number of LCH samples analyzed by whole-exome sequencing is still small, they are consistently found to have a small number of single nucleotide variants, insertions, or deletions compared with other solid tumors that are ERK-driven, such as melanoma.[28,29] Translocations or copy number changes involving relevant loci could provide additional mechanisms for ERK pathway activation. Although recurrent abnormalities of these types have not yet been described in LCH, it is not clear if the technical quality of the assessments performed to date have been sufficiently high to rule them out. Epigenetic alterations could also lead to ERK pathway activation, and global, unbiased analyses of LCH samples for such changes are likely to be the next approach taken by many groups. The challenge for epigenetic analyses, as for RNA sequencing analyses, is determining the appropriate control tissue to make comparisons against. It is also possible that ERK pathway activation in some cases may be non–cell autonomous. For example, overexpression of the macrophage colony-stimulating factor (M-CSF) receptor by LCH cells could lead to heightened responses to ambient M-CSF, including constitutive activation of the ERK signaling pathway. Although this mechanism would not be detected by ordinary genomic analyses of LCH cells, overexpression of receptor tyrosine kinases such as the M-CSF receptor would be detected by careful RNAseq analysis.

Although the presence of mutations in RAF and MEK family members in all subtypes of LCH unifies the disease under a single nosologic category, the fact remains that their clinical manifestations vary widely. So far, no correlations have been found between the presence of specific mutations and a variety of clinical attributes or outcomes other than a higher prevalence of *BRAF* mutations in patients who relapse.[16] Larger numbers of samples drawn from specific clinical subtypes of LCH will have to be analyzed for a larger variety of alterations, including those mentioned earlier, to uncover a possible genomic basis for their disparate clinical behaviors.

The hallmark of treating ERK pathway–driven solid tumors with single-agent RAF inhibitors has been the induction of a profound clinical response followed within a few months by regrowth of the tumor. In contrast, although the number of patients with LCH treated with vemurafenib and reported in the literature is small, they all experienced a clinical benefit from RAF inhibition for as long as they were being treated.[17,52,53] It is striking that there are no reports yet of the development of resistance; this is also the experience reported from the treatment of a larger number of patients with ECD.[53]

One of the main differences between LCH (or ECD) and cancers such as melanoma is the low frequency of genomic alterations in the former compared with the latter. This finding is likely a reflection of genomic stability in LCH, which reduces the probability that LCH cells will generate daughter cells with resistance to RAF inhibitors. This scenario is reminiscent of chronic myelogenous leukemia in which BCR-ABL is the sole driver in most cases and treatment with imatinib can be effective for many years before resistance appears.[55] It remains to be seen how long patients with LCH can be treated with RAF inhibitors without developing resistance, but, for now, it seems that closest therapeutic analog of LCH may be chronic myelogenous leukemia.

REFERENCES

1. Abla O, Egeler RM, Weitzman S. Langerhans cell histiocytosis: current concepts and treatments. Cancer Treat Rev 2010;36(4):354–9.
2. Badalian-Very G, Vergilio JA, Fleming M, et al. Pathogenesis of Langerhans cell histiocytosis. Annu Rev Pathol 2013;8:1–20.
3. Egeler RM, van Halteren AG, Hogendoorn PC, et al. Langerhans cell histiocytosis: fascinating dynamics of the dendritic cell-macrophage lineage. Immunol Rev 2010;234(1):213–32.

4. Guyot-Goubin A, Donadieu J, Barkaoui M, et al. Descriptive epidemiology of childhood Langerhans cell histiocytosis in France, 2000-2004. Pediatr Blood Cancer 2008;51(1):71–5.

5. Stalemark H, Laurencikas E, Karis J, et al. Incidence of Langerhans cell histiocytosis in children: a population-based study. Pediatr Blood Cancer 2008;51(1):76–81.

6. Thomas RK, Baker AC, Debiasi RM, et al. High-throughput oncogene mutation profiling in human cancer. Nat Genet 2007;39(3):347–51.

7. Van Allen EM, Wagle N, Stojanov P, et al. Whole-exome sequencing and clinical interpretation of formalin-fixed, paraffin-embedded tumor samples to guide precision cancer medicine. Nat Med 2014;20(6):682–8.

8. Wagle N, Berger MF, Davis MJ, et al. High-throughput detection of actionable genomic alterations in clinical tumor samples by targeted, massively parallel sequencing. Cancer Discov 2012;2(1):82–93.

9. Badalian-Very G, Vergilio JA, Degar BA, et al. Recurrent BRAF mutations in Langerhans cell histiocytosis. Blood 2010;116(11):1919–23.

10. Davies H, Bignell GR, Cox C, et al. Mutations of the BRAF gene in human cancer. Nature 2002;417(6892):949–54.

11. Garnett MJ, Marais R. Guilty as charged: B-RAF is a human oncogene. Cancer Cell 2004;6(4):313–9.

12. Belden S, Flaherty KT. MEK and RAF inhibitors for BRAF-mutated cancers. Expert Rev Mol Med 2012;14:e17.

13. Samatar AA, Poulikakos PI. Targeting RAS-ERK signalling in cancer: promises and challenges. Nat Rev Drug Discov 2014;13(12):928–42.

14. Hall RD, Kudchadkar RR. BRAF mutations: signaling, epidemiology, and clinical experience in multiple malignancies. Cancer Control 2014;21(3):221–30.

15. Sahm F, Capper D, Preusser M, et al. BRAFV600E mutant protein is expressed in cells of variable maturation in Langerhans cell histiocytosis. Blood 2012;120(12):e28–34.

16. Berres ML, Lim KP, Peters T, et al. BRAF-V600E expression in precursor versus differentiated dendritic cells defines clinically distinct LCH risk groups. J Exp Med 2014;211(4):669–83.

17. Bubolz AM, Weissinger SE, Stenzinger A, et al. Potential clinical implications of BRAF mutations in histiocytic proliferations. Oncotarget 2014;5(12):4060–70.

18. Chilosi M, Facchetti F, Calio A, et al. Oncogene-induced senescence distinguishes indolent from aggressive forms of pulmonary and non-pulmonary Langerhans cell histiocytosis. Leuk Lymphoma 2014;55(11):2620–6.

19. Haroche J, Charlotte F, Arnaud L, et al. High prevalence of BRAF V600E mutations in Erdheim-Chester disease but not in other non-Langerhans cell histiocytoses. Blood 2012;120(13):2700–3.

20. Méhes G, Irsai G, Bedekovics J, et al. Activating BRAF V600E mutation in aggressive pediatric Langerhans cell histiocytosis: demonstration by allele-specific PCR/direct sequencing and immunohistochemistry. Am J Surg Pathol 2014; 38(12):1644–8.

21. Roden AC, Hu X, Kip S, et al. BRAF V600E expression in Langerhans cell histiocytosis: clinical and immunohistochemical study on 25 pulmonary and 54 extrapulmonary cases. Am J Surg Pathol 2014;38(4):548–51.

22. Satoh T, Smith A, Sarde A, et al. B-RAF mutant alleles associated with Langerhans cell histiocytosis, a granulomatous pediatric disease. PLoS One 2012; 7(4):e33891.

23. Varga E, Korom I, Polyanka H, et al. BRAFV600E mutation in cutaneous lesions of patients with adult Langerhans cell histiocytosis. J Eur Acad Dermatol Venereol 2014;29(6):1205–11.

24. Wei R, Wang Z, Li X, et al. Frequent mutation has no effect on tumor invasiveness in patients with Langerhans cell histiocytosis. Biomed Rep 2013;1(3):365–8.

25. Yousem SA, Colby TV, Chen YY, et al. Pulmonary Langerhans' cell histiocytosis: molecular analysis of clonality. Am J Surg Pathol 2001;25(5):630–6.

26. Kansal R, Quintanilla-Martinez L, Datta V, et al. Identification of the V600D mutation in Exon 15 of the BRAF oncogene in congenital, benign Langerhans cell histiocytosis. Genes Chromosomes Cancer 2013;52(1):99–106.

27. Rubinstein JC, Sznol M, Pavlick AC, et al. Incidence of the V600K mutation among melanoma patients with BRAF mutations, and potential therapeutic response to the specific BRAF inhibitor PLX4032. J Transl Med 2010;8:67.

28. Nelson DS, Quispel W, Badalian-Very G, et al. Somatic activating ARAF mutations in Langerhans cell histiocytosis. Blood 2014;123(20):3152–5.

29. Chakraborty R, Hampton OA, Shen X, et al. Mutually exclusive recurrent somatic mutations in MAP2K1 and BRAF support a central role for ERK activation in LCH pathogenesis. Blood 2014;124(19):3007–15.

30. Brown NA, Furtado LV, Betz BL, et al. High prevalence of somatic MAP2K1 mutations in BRAF V600E negative Langerhans cell histiocytosis. Blood 2014;124(10):1655–8.

31. Nelson DS, van Halteren A, Quispel WT, et al. MAP2K1 and MAP3K1 mutations in Langerhans cell histiocytosis. Genes Chromosomes Cancer 2015;54(6):361–8.

32. Hodis E, Watson IR, Kryukov GV, et al. A landscape of driver mutations in melanoma. Cell 2012;150(2):251–63.

33. Marks JL, Gong Y, Chitale D, et al. Novel MEK1 mutation identified by mutational analysis of epidermal growth factor receptor signaling pathway genes in lung adenocarcinoma. Cancer Res 2008;68(14):5524–8.

34. Waterfall JJ, Arons E, Walker RL, et al. High prevalence of MAP2K1 mutations in variant and IGHV4-34-expressing hairy-cell leukemias. Nat Genet 2014;46(1):8–10.

35. Wagle N, Emery C, Berger MF, et al. Dissecting therapeutic resistance to RAF inhibition in melanoma by tumor genomic profiling. J Clin Oncol 2011;29(22):3085–96.

36. Emery CM, Vijayendran KG, Zipser MC, et al. MEK1 mutations confer resistance to MEK and B-RAF inhibition. Proc Natl Acad Sci U S A 2009;106(48):20411–6.

37. Lange-Carter CA, Pleiman CM, Gardner AM, et al. A divergence in the MAP kinase regulatory network defined by MEK kinase and Raf. Science 1993;260(5106):315–9.

38. Ellis MJ, Ding L, Shen D, et al. Whole-genome analysis informs breast cancer response to aromatase inhibition. Nature 2012;486(7403):353–60.

39. Ozono S, Inada H, Nakagawa S, et al. Juvenile myelomonocytic leukemia characterized by cutaneous lesion containing Langerhans cell histiocytosis-like cells. Int J Hematol 2011;93(3):389–93.

40. Diamond EL, Abdel-Wahab O, Pentsova E, et al. Detection of an NRAS mutation in Erdheim-Chester disease. Blood 2013;122(6):1089–91.

41. Emile JF, Diamond EL, Helias-Rodzewicz Z, et al. Recurrent RAS and PIK3CA mutations in Erdheim-Chester disease. Blood 2014;124(19):3016–9.

42. Arceci RJ, Allen CE, Dunkel I, et al. Evaluation of afuresertib, an oral pan-AKT inhibitor, in patients with Langerhans cell histiocytosis. Blood 2013;122(21):2907.

43. Heritier S, Saffroy R, Radosevic-Robin N, et al. Common cancer-associated PIK3CA activating mutations rarely occur in Langerhans cell histiocytosis. Blood 2015;125(15):2448–9.

44. Weintraub M, Bhatia KG, Chandra RS, et al. p53 Expression in Langerhans cell histiocytosis. J Pediatr Hematol Oncol 1998;20(1):12–7.

45. Cao Y, Gao Q, Wazer DE, et al. Abrogation of wild-type p53-mediated transactivation is insufficient for mutant p53-induced immortalization of normal human mammary epithelial cells. Cancer Res 1997;57(24):5584–9.
46. Liu S, Liu XP, El Saddik A. Modeling and distributed gain scheduling strategy for load frequency control in smart grids with communication topology changes. ISA Trans 2014;53(2):454–61.
47. Hinds PW, Finlay CA, Quartin RS, et al. Mutant p53 DNA clones from human colon carcinomas cooperate with ras in transforming primary rat cells: a comparison of the "hot spot" mutant phenotypes. Cell Growth Differ 1990;1(12):571–80.
48. da Costa CE, Szuhai K, van Eijk R, et al. No genomic aberrations in Langerhans cell histiocytosis as assessed by diverse molecular technologies. Genes Chromosomes Cancer 2009;48(3):239–49.
49. Betts DR, Leibundgut KE, Feldges A, et al. Cytogenetic abnormalities in Langerhans cell histiocytosis. Br J Cancer 1998;77(4):552–5.
50. Murakami I, Gogusev J, Fournet JC, et al. Detection of molecular cytogenetic aberrations in Langerhans cell histiocytosis of bone. Hum Pathol 2002;33(5): 555–60.
51. Chikwava KR, Hunt JL, Mantha GS, et al. Analysis of loss of heterozygosity in single-system and multisystem Langerhans' cell histiocytosis. Pediatr Dev Pathol 2007;10(1):18–24.
52. Haroche J, Cohen-Aubart F, Emile JF, et al. Dramatic efficacy of vemurafenib in both multisystemic and refractory Erdheim-Chester disease and Langerhans cell histiocytosis harboring the BRAF V600E mutation. Blood 2013;121(9): 1495–500.
53. Haroche J, Cohen-Aubart F, Emile JF, et al. Reproducible and sustained efficacy of targeted therapy with vemurafenib in patients with BRAF(V600E)-mutated Erdheim-Chester disease. J Clin Oncol 2015;33(5):411–8.
54. Robert C, Karaszewska B, Schachter J, et al. Improved overall survival in melanoma with combined dabrafenib and trametinib. N Engl J Med 2015;372(1):30–9.
55. Druker BJ, Guilhot F, O'Brien SG, et al. Five-year follow-up of patients receiving imatinib for chronic myeloid leukemia. N Engl J Med 2006;355(23):2408–17.

Clinical Characteristics and Treatment of Langerhans Cell Histiocytosis

Chalinee Monsereenusorn, MD[a],
Carlos Rodriguez-Galindo, MD[a,b],*

KEYWORDS

- Langerhans cell histiocytosis • Neurodegeneration • Oncogenes • BRAF
- Chemotherapy

KEY POINTS

- Langerhans cell histiocytosis (LCH) is a neoplasm of myeloid origin characterized by a clonal proliferation of CD1a+/CD207+ cells. In a little more than half of the cases, *BRAF* mutations, predominantly encoding BRAF V600E, are identified; mutations of other members of the MAPK/ERK pathway, such as *MAP2K1* or *ARAF*, are present in another 10% to 25%.
- LCH affects individuals of all ages, although infants more often present with multisystem disease. The disease can affect many tissues and organs of the head and neck. Bony lesions are most common; but the skin, lymph nodes, and brain can also be involved.
- Patients with involvement of only one organ system can often be treated with surgery alone and have excellent outcomes. Patients with multisystem disease, especially with risk-organ involvement, need multimodality treatment and have variable prognoses.
- Treatment with BRAF inhibitors has shown to induce complete and durable responses, and the role of BRAF and MEK inhibitors is currently being investigated.
- LCH neurodegeneration, a devastating long-term complication of LCH, represents one of the major challenges in clinical and translational research of LCH.

INTRODUCTION

Langerhans cell histiocytosis (LCH) is a disease characterized by clonal proliferation of CD1a+/CD207+ myeloid dendritic cells that presents at all ages and with different degrees of systemic involvement. Almost any organ can be affected, and the clinical presentation reflects the tissue-specific inflammatory phenomena. For several

[a] Department of Pediatric Oncology, Dana-Farber/Boston Children's Cancer and Blood Disorders Center, 450 Brookline Avenue D3-133, Boston, MA 02215, USA; [b] Department of Pediatrics, Harvard Medical School, Boston, MA, USA
* Corresponding author. Dana-Farber/Boston Children's Cancer and Blood Disorders Center, 450 Brookline Avenue D3-133, Boston MA 02215.
E-mail address: carlos_rodriguez-galindo@dfci.harvard.edu

decades, LCH has been considered to be a reactive clonal proliferation of Langerhans cells; however, in recent years, LCH has been defined as a neoplasm of myeloid origin, with a significant inflammatory component that defines some of the acute and long-term manifestations. This evolution from an immune disorder to a neoplasia has reframed the disease and opened the door for the development of targeted therapies.

BIOLOGY

The pathogenic cells are known to originate from a myeloid-derived precursor and are uniformly characterized by activation of the MAPK/ERK signaling pathway; ERK activation is documented in all cases.[1,2] In up to two-thirds of cases, pathway activation is secondary to a somatic mutation in *BRAF (BRAF[V600E])*; in other cases, mutations in *MAP2K1*[3] or less frequently in other members of the pathway, such as *ARAF*,[4] have been described. About one-quarter of cases have no known genomic abnormalities.

EPIDEMIOLOGY

The estimated incidence of LCH is 8.9 cases per million children younger than 15 years per year, with a median age at diagnosis of 3 years old.[5] The causes and risk factors for developing LCH are unclear.[6] However, the unique patterns of presentation, ranging from localized bone lesions with spontaneous regression to disseminated forms with multiorgan involvement, suggest a complex pathogenesis. Familial associations, particularly the observation of increased incidence in monozygotic twins of affected patients, have suggested the presence of a germline predisposition at least for a proportion of cases.[7] Also, population-based studies have shown differences in the incidence of disseminated LCH by race and ethnic group; a higher incidence has been reported for Hispanics and a lower incidence for blacks.[8] Studies have also shown a correlation with maternal and neonatal infections,[6,9,10] lack of childhood vaccinations,[6,9] family history of thyroid disease,[6] in vitro fertilization,[11] and feeding problems and transfusions during infancy.[10] Finally, lower socioeconomic conditions have been associated with an increased incidence of disseminated LCH.[8]

PATHOLOGY

Since pathologic Langerhans cells activate other immunologic cells, microscopic examination of diseased tissue shows eosinophils, neutrophils, lymphocytes, and histiocytes in addition to the LCH cells; this appearance is what has been traditionally described as eosinophilic granuloma. Abscesses and necrosis may be present. LCH cells are large, oval , and mononuclear, with a prominent nucleus and eosinophilic cytoplasm. They do not have dendritic cell processes like cutaneous Langerhans cells. They stain positive for protein S-100, CD1a, and CD207 (langerin) and contain cytoplasmic rod-shaped inclusions called Birbeck granules. A diagnosis of LCH is made by typical positive staining with CD1a or CD207.[12]

With the development of new technology for accurate detection of cell-free DNA, *BRAF[V600E]* mutation analysis in plasma and urine has shown to be an effective tool for diagnosis and monitoring of disease activity in patients with LCH.[13]

CLINICAL PRESENTATION

Classically, LCH was defined as 3 distinct diseases; eosinophilic granuloma, Hand-Schüller-Christian disease, and Abt-Letterer-Siwe disease were different clinical descriptions within the same spectrum of progressive system involvement. *Eosinophilic granuloma*, whether solitary or multifocal, is found predominantly in older children as well as in young adults, with a peak incidence between 5 and 10 years of age. Eosinophilic granuloma is the most common form of LCH, accounting for approximately 60% to 80% of the diagnoses. *Hand-Schüller-Christian disease* was historically described as a clinical triad of lytic bone lesions, exophthalmos caused by orbital involvement, and diabetes insipidus (DI). It is most commonly described in the first 4 to 7 years of life, and it may account for approximately 15% to 40% of all LCH cases. *Abt-Letterer-Siwe disease* is the most severe manifestation of LCH, albeit rare. Typically, patients are less than 2 years of age and present with a scaly seborrheic rash, ear discharge, and signs of severe systemic involvement with symptoms such as cytopenias, pulmonary dysfunction, lymphadenopathy, or hepatosplenomegaly.[14] Nowadays, this old terminology has been replaced by a classification system that is based on the site of lesions, number of involved sites (single or multisystem/local or multifocal), and whether the disease involves risk organs (hematopoietic system, liver, or spleen). This classification is the basis for the risk-adapted treatment used in the LCH-III protocol discussed later (**Table 1**).

SITES OF INVOLVEMENT

All organs can be affected by LCH; therefore, a comprehensive evaluation is indicated. The most commonly involved organs and systems are highlighted next:

Bone

Bone is the most commonly affected system; bone lesions are present in approximately 80% of patients with LCH.[15] The most common site of involvement is the skull (27%), followed by the femur (13%), mandible (11%), and pelvis (10%).[16] Mostly, radiographic studies typically show lytic lesions, especially punched-out lesions in the skull without marginal sclerosis or periosteal reaction (**Fig. 1**). Pain and tumor formation in a localized area of bone is a very common presentation of LCH. In the skull, the lesions are usually soft and tender to touch. Skull lesions may include a soft tissue mass pressing on the dura, but severe intracranial extension is rare. Involvement of the skull base is also very common in LCH; typical locations include the bones of the orbit or the temporal bone (typically the mastoid). In these cases, otitis media or externa are common presenting signs. Involvement of the vertebral bodies is also common, and the presence of a vertebra plana is frequent.

Table 1
Clinical classification of patients with LCH according to the Histiocyte Society LCH-III Trial

Clinical Group	Involved System	Involved Organs
1	Multisystem risk patients	Any risk[a] organ involvement
2	Multisystem low-risk patients	≥2 Organ *without* risk[a] organ involvement
3	Single system • Multifocal or • Special site[b]	≥2 Lesions in *one* organ or in special site[b]
—	Single system Unifocal or localized	1 Lesion in one organ

[a] Risk organs consist of lung, liver, spleen, bone marrow, or hematological dysfunction.
[b] Special sites are intracranial soft tissue extension or vertebral lesions with intraspinal soft tissue extension.
Adapted from Gadner H, Minkov M, Grois N, et al. Therapy prolongation improves outcome in multisystem Langerhans cell histiocytosis. Blood 2013;121(25):5006–14.

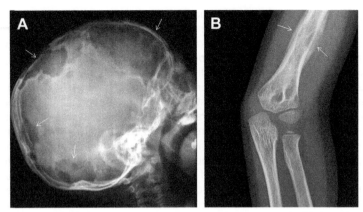

Fig. 1. Typical appearance of eosinophilic granulomas (*arrows*) in the skull (*A*) and humerus (*B*).

Skin

The most common skin lesions are seborrheic eczema, which typically occurs in infants, and a neonatal form characterized by disseminated brown to red papules with common central ulceration (**Fig. 2**). Isolated skin involvement usually carries a good prognosis, with approximately 60% chance of regression. However, close

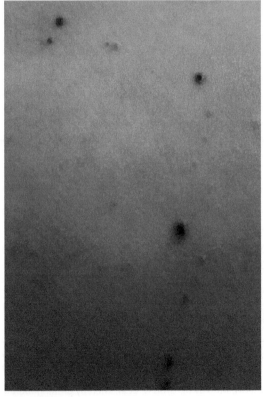

Fig. 2. Neonatal cutaneous LCH.

monitoring is required, as reactivation or progression to multisystem involvement has been observed in up to 40% of cases.[12,17]

Neuroendocrine and Central Nervous Systems

DI caused by involvement of the pituitary stalk occurs in approximately 25% of cases, usually after therapy. LCH is also a common diagnosis in patients with DI of unknown cause, and almost all patients with DI caused by LCH have involvement of other organs concurrently or subsequently.[14] Anterior pituitary involvement, commonly represented by growth hormone deficiency, is also a common complication and highlights the importance of a comprehensive endocrine monitoring in patients with LCH. Mass lesions of the gray or white matter are less frequent (1%). Involvement of the sphenoid, orbital, ethmoid, zygomatic, or temporal bones confers a higher (25% overall) risk for central nervous system (CNS) involvement (CNS-risk lesions), including late neurodegeneration (see later discussion), an inflammatory phenomenon of unclear pathogenesis that is characterized by cerebellar dysfunction and neurocognitive deficits.[18]

Pulmonary

Involvement of the lungs usually occurs in the context of multisystem involvement, commonly limited to young children. Patients usually present with pulmonary dysfunction including tachypnea, dyspnea, and cough. Radiographic findings are typical for the presence of a reticulonodular pattern with bullae formation. Isolated pulmonary involvement is a rare presentation that is almost exclusively found in adults with a smoking habit (discussed later).[19]

Hematopoietic System

The presence of hematopoietic dysfunction in the form of cytopenias is a poor prognostic sign. It occurs in the context of multisystem involvement, more frequently in young children. Its pathophysiology is multifactorial, including direct involvement of the bone marrow as well as peripheral destruction caused by hypersplenism from Langerhans cell infiltrates in the spleen.[20]

Hepatobiliary System

Liver involvement, which typically occurs in infants with multisystem disease, also carries a poor prognosis. Patients present with hypoalbuminemia, edema, hepatomegaly, or conjugated hyperbilirubinemia. A well-described complication of hepatic involvement is the development of sclerosing cholangitis and hepatic fibrosis, which can result in liver failure and need for liver transplantation.[14]

TREATMENT OF LANGERHANS CELL HISTIOCYTOSIS

The treatment of LCH over the years has reflected the changing concepts of the disease process. Indeed, the difficulties in developing more effective therapies are linked to the deficiencies in the understanding of the pathogenesis of LCH. Retrospective studies of Lahey[21] and Komp and colleagues[22] showed that, although many organs can harbor proliferating pathogenic cells, only if organ function was disrupted was such involvement of prognostic significance. Patients could then be stratified into different risk categories based on the extent of their disease and the degree of organ dysfunction. Patients with single-system disease confined to a single site usually require only local therapy or observation. Patients with more extensive disease require systemic therapy; several groups have explored risk-based approaches, which are summarized next.

Histiocyte Society's Langerhans Cell Histiocytosis Studies

Langerhans Cell Histiocytosis-I (LCH-I)

The first international randomized trial for multisystem LCH (MS-LCH), LCH-I (1991–1995), randomized patients to receive weekly vinblastine or etoposide every 3 weeks for 24 weeks. Overall survival was close to 80%, with no significant differences by treatment arm. Involvement of the hematopoietic system, lung, liver, and spleen, age at diagnosis less than 2 years old, and poor response at 6 weeks were significantly associated with an adverse outcome.[23] In comparison with the contemporaneous DAL-HX 83 study, which explored a more intensive and longer regimen, LCH-I showed a lower 6-week response rate (50% vs 80%) and a higher reactivation rate (50% vs 30%).[24]

Langerhans Cell Histiocytosis-II (LCH-II)

The LCH-II study (1996–2001) followed on the LCH-I findings and explored early intensification through a randomized design that investigated the addition of etoposide (arm B) to a standard 6-week induction with prednisone and vinblastine and continuation with 6-mercaptopurine and every-3-week pulses of prednisone and vinblastine for a total of 24 weeks of therapy (arm A).[25] Both arms produced similar outcomes in terms of 6-week response rates (63% arm A vs 71% arm B), 5-year survival probability (74% vs 79%), and disease reactivation rates (46% both arms); however, the more intensive arm B resulted in reduced mortality for patients with risk organ involvement. The LCH-II study also showed that patients younger than 2 years without risk-organ involvement have excellent response rates and a 100% survival, and patients with risk-organ involvement and poor response at 6 weeks have the highest mortality.[25] Those findings helped refine the risk-stratification and treatment for its successor study, the LCH-III.

Langerhans Cell Histiocytosis-III (LCH-III)

The LCH-III study (2001–2008) was built following a risk-adapted model with the main objectives of investigating the impact of the addition of methotrexate on the outcome of patients with risk-organ involvement and the effect of therapy prolongation on decreasing the incidence of disease reactivation for patients with multisystem disease.[26] The 3 risk groups are depicted in **Table 1**. Patients with MS-LCH with risk-organ involvement (group 1) received standard induction with prednisone and vinblastine and continuation with the same drugs with the addition of 6-mercaptopurine for a total duration of 12 months and were randomized to the addition of methotrexate; patients with active disease at 6 weeks received a modified reinduction (**Fig. 3**). The outcome was similar in both arms, with a 5-year survival probability of 84%, response rates of 71%, and reactivation rates of 27%. Historical comparisons revealed superior outcomes compared with LCH-I and LCH-II in terms of survival and reactivation rates. The 3-year cumulative incidence of DI was also similar in both arms (8% in standard arm and 9% in methotrexate arm).[26]

The outcome for patients with MS-LCH without risk-organ involvement is excellent, with survival rates close to 100% across studies. However, in the LCH-I and LCH-II studies, almost half of these patients sustained a disease reactivation. Based on the lower reactivation rates noted in the DAL-HX-83 study, which prolonged treatment for 12 months, the LCH-III protocol investigated the effect of treatment duration for this group of patients (group 2) and randomized them to a standard regimen of vinblastine and prednisone for 6 or 12 months (**Fig. 4**). Longer treatment resulted in a significantly lower 5-year reactivation rate (37% vs 54%, P = .03). The 3-year cumulative incidence of DI was 12% in both arms.[26]

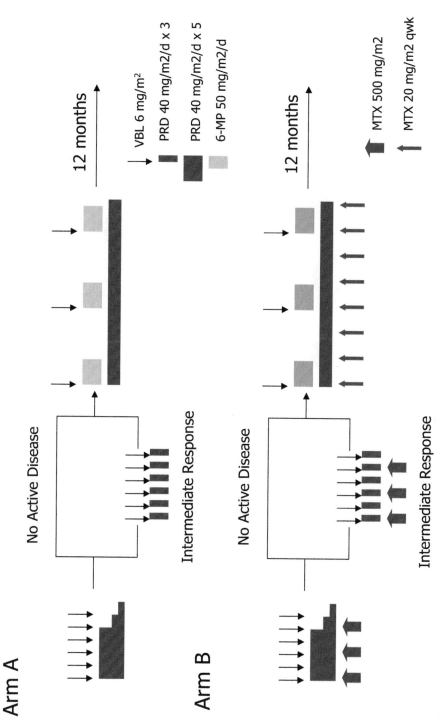

Fig. 3. LCH-III protocol: Treatment of patients with multisystem disease and risk-organ involvement (group 1). intermed, intermediate. MP, 6-mercaptopurine; MTX, methotrexate; PRD, prednisone; VBL, vinblastine.

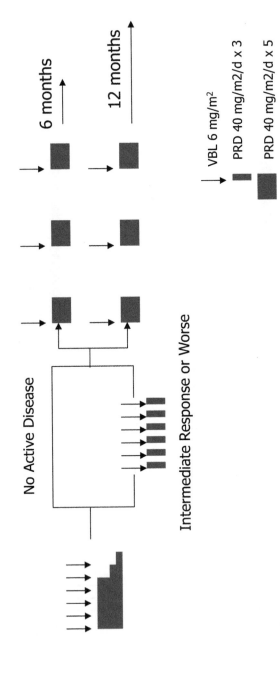

Fig. 4. LCH-III protocol: Treatment of patients with multisystem disease without risk-organ involvement (group 2).

Group 3 included patients with single-system multifocal disease (mostly multifocal bone) and patients with single bone lesions in special sites. Special sites were defined as involvement of the craniofacial bones with intracranial extension and patients with vertebral lesions with intraspinal soft tissue extension. Those patients were treated with a standard 6-month regimen of prednisone and vinblastine.

Langerhans Cell Histiocytosis-IV

The LCH-IV protocol represents a major international effort to integrate the most relevant clinical questions in a prospective trial, of which the overarching objectives are as follows: (1) to improve survival for patients with risk-organ involvement by early switching to intensive nucleoside-analogue–based therapy; (2) to investigate whether further prolongation of therapy will decrease reactivation rates; and (3) to investigate the incidence, pathogenesis, and treatment of LCH-induced neurodegeneration. Thus, the LCH-IV study provides an excellent framework on which major therapeutic questions can be addressed. Because of the extreme complexity of the disease presentations and course scenarios, the LCH-IV study consists of 7 strata:

Stratum I This stratum includes the first-line treatment of patients with MS LCH (group 1) and patients with single-system (SS) LCH with multifocal bone or CNS-risk lesions (group 2). Group 1 patients will undergo a double randomization; all will receive a standard prednisone/vinblastine regimen and will be randomized to 12 versus 24 months and to the addition of 6-mercaptopurine. Group 2 patients will be randomized to receive the standard prednisone/vinblastine regimen for 6 versus 12 months.

Stratum II This stratum includes the second-line treatment of nonrisk patients (patients without risk-organ involvement who fail first-line therapy or have a reactivation after completion of first-line therapy). Patients will be treated with a combination of vincristine and low-dose cytarabine (ara-C) for 24 weeks, after which they will be randomized to indomethacin or a combination of oral 6-mercaptopurine and methotrexate as maintenance.

Stratum III This stratum includes salvage treatment of risk LCH (patients with dysfunction of risk organs who fail first-line therapy). This group of patients with high-risk disease has the worse outcome; in order to improve survival, an early switch (in first 6 weeks) to this salvage arm will be indicated. Treatment includes an intense regimen based on high-dose cytarabine and cladribine.

Stratum IV This stratum includes stem cell transplantation for risk LCH (patients with dysfunction of risk organs who fail first-line therapy).

Stratum V This stratum includes monitoring and treatment of isolated tumorous and neurodegenerative CNS-LCH. This stratum will study the efficacy of cladribine in isolated tumorous CNS-LCH and intravenous immunoglobulin and cytarabine in neurodegenerative CNS-LCH treatment.

Stratum VI This stratum includes the natural history and management of other SS-LCH (patients who do not need systemic therapy at the time of diagnosis).

Stratum VII This stratum includes the long-term follow-up. (All patients irrespective of previous therapy will be followed for reactivation or permanent consequences once complete disease resolution has been achieved and the respective protocol treatment completed.)

The definition of risk organ involvement is depicted in **Box 1**; importantly, in LCH-IV, lung involvement is no longer considered an adverse prognostic factor as it was in earlier studies.[27]

DAL-HX Studies

The DAL-HX 83 and DAL-HX 90 studies were conducted between 1983 and 1991 by 62 institutions in Austria, Germany, Switzerland, and the Netherlands and applied a risk-adapted treatment. Three groups of patients were defined by multifocal bone disease (group A), soft tissue involvement without organ dysfunction (group B), and organ dysfunction (group C). All patients received a 6-week induction regimen with prednisone, vinblastine, and etoposide and continuation with oral 6-mercaptopurine and pulses of prednisone and vinblastine, with the addition of etoposide for group B patients and etoposide and methotrexate for group C patients. Approximately 90% of group A and B patients and 70% of group C patients achieved a complete response, for an overall survival at 5 years of 81%.[28,29]

Japan Langerhans Cell Histiocytosis Study Group and the Role Cytarabine

The Japan LCH Study Group-96 (JLSG-96) protocol (1996–2001) was a nonrandomized response-based trial with a cytarabine backbone that represents an interesting alternative to the prednisone/vinblastine regimens explored in the Histiocyte Society's studies.[30] Patients received a 6-week induction with cytarabine, vincristine, and prednisolone, which had been shown to be effective in a Dutch study previously.[31] Responding patients subsequently received a 24-week maintenance phase alternating cytarabine, vincristine, and prednisolone with methotrexate and prednisolone. Poor responders to induction treatment were switched to an alternative induction phase with doxorubicin, cyclophosphamide, vincristine, and prednisolone and subsequently continued to receive alternating cycles of those agents as maintenance.[30] This regimen resulted in excellent response rates (96.9% in multisite SS-LCH and 78.0% in MS-LCH). DI developed in 3.1% of patients in the single-system group and in 8.9% of patients in the MS-LCH group. The overall survival rates at 5 years for

---

Box 1
Definition of risk organ involvement in LCH-IV

Hematopoietic involvement: (with or without bone marrow involvement[a])

At least 2 of the following:

1. *Anemia:* hemoglobin less than 100 g/L (<10 g/dL), infants less than 90 g/L (<9.0 g/dL), not from other causes (eg, iron deficiency)

2. *Leukocytopenia:* leukocytes less than 4.0×10^9/L (4000/μL)

3. *Thrombocytopenia:* platelets less than 100×10^9/L (100.000/μL)

Spleen involvement: enlargement greater than 2 cm below costal margin in the midclavicular line[b]

Liver involvement: one or more of the following

1. *Enlargement* greater than 3 cm below costal margin in the midclavicular line[b]

2. *Dysfunction* (ie, hypoproteinemia <55 g/L, hypoalbuminemia <25 g/L, not from other causes)

3. *Histopathologic findings* of active disease

[a] Bone marrow involvement is defined as presence of CD1a-positive cells on marrow slides.
[b] Enlargement in *centimeters below the costal margin* as assessed by physical examination.

the single-system and MS groups were 100% and 94.4% ±3.2%, respectively; reactivation rates were 28.1% for single-system and 45.3% for MS.[30] The good results of this cytarabine-based regimen have provided the rationale for the low-risk salvage regimen in LCH-IV and have prompted the proposal to consider cytarabine as a good alternative to vinblastine and prednisolone for front-line treatment of LCH.[32]

Because of the high reactivation rates in JLSG-96, the successor study JLSG-02 was adapted to increase the cumulative dose of prednisolone during induction, to add cyclosporin A to the regimen for poor responders, and to increase the duration of continuation therapy with the addition of 6-mercaptopurine, vinblastine, prednisolone, and methotrexate for an additional 18 weeks, increasing the total duration of treatment to 12 months. Preliminary results showed an increase in the initial response rates and a decrease in disease reactivation for patients with MS-LCH.[33]

The outcomes of the studies discussed earlier are summarized in **Table 2**.

TREATMENT OF RECURRENT LANGERHANS CELL HISTIOCYTOSIS

Disease reactivation is common in patients with LCH; depending on the duration of the front-line treatment, 20% to 50% of patients may experience a relapse. In general terms, 2 groups of patients are identified:

1. Patients with low-risk disease: This group includes patients with reactivation of multifocal bone disease or low-risk multisystem disease (without risk organ involvement); disease reactivations occur in approximately one-third of patients, and they usually respond well to second-line therapy. Many regimens have been described, including oral 6-mercaptopurine and methotrexate,[34] indomethacin,[35,36] bisphosphonates,[37] BRAF inhibitors,[38] and nucleoside analogues, such as cladribine, cytarabine, and clofarabine.[39–41]

2. Patients with high-risk disease: This high-risk group is characterized by the presence of risk organ involvement and poor response to standard treatment. Mortality is high, and recent data suggest that an intense regimen with cladribine and high-dose cytarabine may be effective.[42] Allogeneic hematopoietic stem cell transplantation

Table 2
Comparison of outcomes among different LCH protocols

| Variable | Multifocal SS-LCH | | | MS-LCH | | | | | LCH-III | |
	DAL-HX	JLSG-96	JLSG-02	DAL-HX	JLSG-96	JLSG-02	LCH-I	LCH-II	RO −	RO +
N	34	32	67	63	59	97	143	193	269	285
Duration (mo)	12	7.5	12	12	7.5	12	6	6	6/12	12
Response rate (%)	94.1	96.9	85.1	79	76.3	84.5	53	67	86	70–72
Reactivation rate (%)	17.6	28.1	22	30	45.3	25	58	46	54/37	25–29
Survival rate (%)	—	100	100	94	94.4	97.6	79	76.5	99	84
Incidence of DI (%)	2.9	3.2	1.5	11.9	8.9	18.6	22.5	21.8	12	8–9

Abbreviation: RO, risk organ.

has also been proposed for those cases.[43] BRAF inhibitors may also play a role in the treatment of this group of patients.

2-Chlorodeoxyadenosine (Cladribine)

The analogue 2-chlorodeoxyadenosine (cladribine) is a purine analogue that in children has mainly been used in the treatment of acute myeloid leukemia, whereby responses of up to 59% are obtained as a single agent.[44] Excellent clinical responses, with an overall response rate of 82%, were initially reported in adults with recurrent LCH.[45] This finding prompted the study of this agent further in children with recurrent LCH. For patients with low-risk disease reactivation, cladribine (5 mg/m^2/d × 5 days) has shown to induce responses in greater than 90% of the patients, although further reactivations still occur.[39,46–48] One additional benefit of cladribine is its effect on CNS disease.[49] A major problem with the use of cladribine is its limitation to a short treatment course; more than 4 or 6 courses of treatment are associated with prolonged myelosuppression, causing a clinical picture similar to myelodysplasia. For patients with high-risk disease, cladribine as a single agent has little effect,[47] and a more intensive regimen is needed. The combination of higher dosages of cladribine (9 mg/m^2/d × 5 days) with cytarabine (1 g/m^2/d × 5 days) has induced complete responses in patients with refractory disease.[42,50] Although this treatment is effective, it is associated with high morbidity, with treatment-related mortality in excess of 20%. Recent data suggest that a lower-dosage regimen (cytarabine 100 mg/m^2/d × 5 days with cladribine 5 mg/m^2/d × 5 days) may also be effective in this group of patients with high-risk disease.[51]

Clofarabine

Clofarabine is a second-generation deoxyadenosine analogue with documented efficacy in the treatment of children with relapsed acute lymphoblastic leukemia and acute myeloid leukemia.[52,53] Given the good results obtained with cladribine in the management of recurrent LCH, there could be a role for the use of this agent in this same population. Clofarabine monotherapy at dosages of 25 to 30 mg/m^2/d × 5 days has shown to induce significant responses, including patients with MS-LCH with risk-organ involvement and patients with refractory disease to cladribine and cytarabine.[40,41,54] Moreover, clofarabine has demonstrated activity against juvenile xanthogranuloma and Rosai–Dorfman disease.[41]

Cytarabine

Cytarabine, alone or in combination with corticosteroids or vincristine, has shown efficacy against refractory LCH, particularly in cases with CNS disease.[31,55] Dosages of 100 to 150 mg/m^2/d × 5 days have been typically used, and toxicity seems to be low.[55] Cytarabine at varying doses (100 mg to 1 g/m^2/d × 5 days) has been used in combination with cladribine for the treatment of patients with refractory LCH with risk-organ involvement (see earlier discussion).[42,51]

Bisphosphonates

Bisphosphonates are pyrophosphate analogues that inhibit the recruitment of osteoclasts and reduce their activity and durability. Pamidronate has been used for the treatment of bony lesions in patients without involvement of risk organs. Given at a dosage of 1 mg/kg every 4 weeks for 6 doses, the 3-year progression-free survival was 56.3% ±12.4%.[37] The outcome was significantly better in children with a first reactivation compared with second or subsequent reactivations. The results of this study underline the efficacy of bisphosphonates for the treatment of bony recurrent LCH, although prospective trials are needed to confirm the efficacy and safety of bisphosphonates in this condition.[56] Zoledronic acid has also shown to be effective in adults with multifocal bone disease.[57]

Indomethacin

Prostaglandins have been implicated in the pathogenesis of the bone lesions in LCH.[35] Treatment with indomethacin at dosages of 1 to 2 mg/kg/d given for a median of 4 months has shown to induce responses and regression of bone lesions in more than 90% of patients with symptomatic single-system bone lesions, either at diagnosis or at the time of relapse.[36] These findings provide the rationale for the use of this agent in the treatment of low-risk reactivations proposed in LCH-IV.

BRAF Inhibitors

The presence of the oncogenic *BRAF* V600E mutation in up to two-thirds of patients, as well as its association with an increased risk of reactivation, provides a very strong rationale for the use of BRAF inhibitors.[58] The *BRAF* V600E gain-of-function mutations have also been observed in a large proportion of patients with Erdheim-Chester disease (ECD).[59] Vemurafenib has been reported to induce significant responses in patients with multisystem and refractory ECD and LCH carrying the *BRAF* V600E mutation.[38,60] Contrary to what has been observed with other malignancies, no drug resistance has been reported.[60] Given the universal activation of the MAPK pathway regardless of *BRAF* mutational status, the role of MEK inhibitors in the treatment of LCH is currently being explored.

Imatinib Mesylate

Imatinib mesylate has shown an inhibitory effect on differentiation of CD34+ progenitor cells into dendritic cells, thus providing some rationale for its use in histiocytic disorders. Clinical and radiological responses have been observed in adult patients with LCH and ECD either as first- or second-line treatment.[61]

Hematopoietic Stem Cell Transplantation

Despite progress made in the treatment of LCH, a significant proportion of patients with risk-organ involvement fail to respond to standard or first-line salvage regimens. Hematopoietic stem cell transplantation may provide an effective alternative through high-dose chemotherapy, replacement of stem cells, generation of a graft-versus-LCH effect, and immunomodulation. In one study, the 10-year overall survival for patients with risk-organ involvement at diagnosis was 50%.[62] Because of the previous treatment-related effects, reduced intensity conditioning regimens are a preferable procedure with low transplant-related morbidity and mortality.[43]

SPECIAL CONSIDERATIONS
Adult Langerhans Cell Histiocytosis

The rarity of LCH in adults combined with the nonspecific and varied clinical presentations typically result in missed and delayed diagnoses.[63,64] Adult LCH usually presents after the fourth decade, and most patients have multisystem involvement at diagnosis. In 6% of the cases, patients have been diagnosed with other neoplastic diseases. The lung is the organ most frequently involved; this presentation, either alone or as part of multisystem disease, is strongly associated with a smoking habit.[65] In general, the clinical presentation and organs involved are similar to pediatric patients, with more frequent involvement of the genitalia, particularly in women.[66]

Treatment of LCH in adults generally follows similar guidelines as pediatric LCH but with some modifications.[63] The more severe skin manifestations have shown to respond well to phototherapy[67] and low-dose methotrexate.[68] For patients requiring systemic therapy, the adverse side effects associated with corticosteroid therapy and vinblastine may limit treatment compliance; for this reason, treatment with cytarabine or cladribine is generally preferred,[63,69] although BRAF inhibitors are being increasingly used in this population.[38]

Pulmonary Langerhans Cell Histiocytosis

Lung involvement in children with LCH usually presents in the context of multisystem disease. In contrast, pulmonary involvement in adults usually occurs in isolation; it is strongly associated with cigarette smoking, typically in the third to fifth decades of life.[19] The frequency of *BRAF* V600E mutations in lung lesions of LCH in adult patients is lower (less than one-third of the cases), but the presence of the mutation seems to be associated with the cumulative tobacco exposure.[70] The clinical presentation of pulmonary LCH is usually a nonspecific dry cough; the interval between the onset of clinical symptoms and diagnosis varies but is approximately 6 months. The most common finding on chest radiography is the presence of a reticulo-micronodular infiltration, with cyst formation in more advanced cases. High-resolution computed tomography is required for better diagnosis; typical findings are the presence of small, often cavitated nodules and thin-wall cysts. Pulmonary function test usually show reduced carbon monoxide diffusing capacity in 70% to 90% of the patients. The gold standard for diagnosis is lung biopsy and the identification of activated pathogenic LCH cells in loose granulomas. The natural history of pulmonary LCH is widely variable; smoking cessation is mandatory for improving, and up to 50% of the patients experience a favorable outcome either spontaneously or with a short course of steroids.[19] Patients with suboptimal responses after smoking cessation and steroid therapy may benefit from treatment with cladribine.[63,71] In cases of advanced disease, lung transplantation may be required.[72]

Central Nervous System Langerhans Cell Histiocytosis

CNS involvement may present in different forms and over a long period of time, representing a spectrum of diseases ranging from active infiltration by LCH to long-term effects. The classic clinical presentation is diabetes insipidus[18]; however, with the wide use of advanced neuroimaging, CNS alterations in patients with LCH are more frequent than previously thought.[73] The risk factors for CNS-LCH include the presence of CNS-risk lesions and extended disease activity.[18] The clinical presentation of CNS-LCH depends on the site and type of CNS involvement. DI, the most common presentation, is the hallmark of hypothalamic pituitary involvement, which has been found in 25% of all patients with LCH and in up to 50% of patients with MS-LCH.[74,75] Growth hormone deficiency is the second most common endocrinopathy, and it occurs in up to 50% of patients with LCH with DI.[76] Prolonged systemic therapy seems to be associated with a lower incidence of endocrinopathies; in the most recent studies, the incidence of DI in patients with MS-LCH is approximately 10%.[26] Patients with tumorous lesions may present with headache, seizures, focal neurologic deficits, or signs and symptoms of increased intracranial pressure. A not-yet-well-quantified proportion of patients with a history of LCH develop a progressive neurodegenerative disease. This risk is up to 10% in patients with DI.[75] Some asymptomatic patients may have typical MRI changes of radiologic neurodegeneration for years; however, others have clinical neurodegeneration, including subtle tremor, abnormal reflexes, gait disturbance, motor spasticity, ataxia, dysarthria, dysphagia, behavioral changes, learning disorders, or psychiatric problems.[18] The management of patients with CNS-LCH consists of a complete neurologic examination, neuropsychological testing, endocrine and ophthalmologic evaluation, and neuroimaging. Brain biopsy is only indicated for patients without an established diagnosis of LCH who have a negative diagnostic workup for extracranial LCH lesions.

The most crucial investigative tool for CNS involvement by LCH is MRI. The classification of MRI findings in CNS-LCH identifies 3 groups: tumorous/granulomatous, nontumorous/nongranulomatous, and atrophy lesions (**Box 2**).[18] In tumorous lesions, the MRI typically shows space-occupying tumors with or without calcification; the more common form is in the hypothalamic-pituitary axis, where an enlargement of the pituitary stalk is found. When DI develops, a loss of the bright spot in the posterior pituitary is a common finding. In nontumorous lesions, the findings include symmetric hyperintense signal changes on T2-weighted imaging and hypointense or hyperintense signals on T1-weighted imaging (T1WI) in the cerebellar gray matter extending to the surrounding white matter or presenting as cerebellar atrophy. In the basal

---

Box 2
Classification of MRI finding in patients with CNS LCH

Tumorous/granulomatous lesions

- Granulomatous lesions of skull bones
- Hypothalamic pituitary region (most common site)
- Posterior pituitary
- Anterior pituitary
- Pituitary stalk
- Hypothalamus
- Pineal gland
- Choroid plexus
- Meninges
- Enhancing parenchymal lesions

Nontumorous/nongranulomatous intracerebral lesions

- Dentate nucleus[a]
- Cerebellar white matter[a]
- Basal ganglia[a]
- Brainstem, pons[a]
- Supratentorial white matter
- Virchow-Robin spaces

Atrophy

- Cerebellar atrophy
- Midbrain atrophy
- Supratentorial atrophy

[a] Radiologic neurodegeneration.

Modified from Grois N, Fahrner B, Arceci RJ, et al. Central nervous system disease in Langerhans cell histiocytosis. J Pediatr 2010;156(6):873–81, 881.e1.

ganglia, the MRI findings include hyperintense signals on T1WI usually involving the globus pallidus. These findings are commonly referred to as radiological neurodegeneration.[18,77] Two other patterns of parenchymal white matter changes include the presence of dilated Virchow-Robin spaces and a leukoencephalopathylike pattern that may involve the cerebellum, pons, and periventricular white matter.[18]

Cerebrospinal fluid studies are not generally recommended in all patients with LCH with CNS symptoms; however, they should be considered in the context of investigation of biomarkers of neurodegeneration. The histopathology of CNS-LCH is not well defined because of the lack of comprehensive studies and limited availability of tissue specimens. In general, 3 histopathologic patterns have been described: (1) circumscribed granulomas with a variable presence of CD1a+ cells and a strong CD8+ T-lymphocytic infiltration; (2) neurodegenerative lesions with negative CD1a and a profound CD8+ inflammatory process, associated with neuronal and axonal degeneration and secondary myelin loss; and (3) granulomas in infundibular tumors invading the hypothalamus with diffuse infiltration of the surrounding CNS parenchyma by CD1a+ histiocytes.[18]

There are no standard guidelines for the treatment of CNS-LCH. For tumorous lesions and new-onset DI, treatment with a standard LCH regimen is indicated; vinblastine and prednisone or single-agent cladribine have shown to be effective.[49,78] Treatment of neurodegenerative disease is less well defined. Improvement in the neurologic condition has been reported with the use of cytarabine[55] and intravenous immunoglobulin.[79] Anecdotal responses or disease stabilization have also been documented with infliximab[80] and cis-retinoic acid.[81] However, a better understanding of the pathophysiology of this syndrome is required to develop more rational treatments.

SUMMARY AND FUTURE DIRECTIONS

LCH is a neoplasm of myeloid origin characterized by activation of the MAPK/ERK pathway and with a wide spectrum of clinical presentations and variable outcomes. With current risk-adapted treatments, more than 80% of patients are cured. However, 30% to 50% of patients experience disease recurrence; a significant number of survivors develop neurodegeneration. Treatments aimed at achieving long-term cures with low reactivation rates and that could prevent the development of neurodegeneration need to be developed. Targeted therapies with BRAF or MEK inhibitors offer the possibility of reframing the treatment of LCH in the near future.

REFERENCES

1. Badalian-Very G, Vergilio JA, Degar BA, et al. Recent advances in the understanding of Langerhans cell histiocytosis. Br J Haematol 2012;156(2):163–72.
2. Allen CE, Li L, Peters TL, et al. Cell-Specific gene expression in Langerhans cell histiocytosis lesions reveals a distinct profile compared with epidermal Langerhans cells. J Immunol 2010;184(8):4557–67.
3. Chakraborty R, Hampton OA, Shen X, et al. Mutually exclusive recurrent somatic mutations in MAP2K1 and BRAF support a central role for ERK activation in LCH pathogenesis. Blood 2014;124(19):3007–15.
4. Nelson DS, Quispel W, Badalian-Very G, et al. Somatic activating ARAF mutations in Langerhans cell histiocytosis. Blood 2014;123(20):3152–5.
5. Stalemark H, Laurencikas E, Karis J, et al. Incidence of Langerhans cell histiocytosis in children: a population-based study. Pediatr Blood Cancer 2008;51(1):76–81.
6. Bhatia S, Nesbit ME Jr, Egeler M, et al. Epidemiologic study of Langerhans cell histiocytosis in children. J Pediatr 1997;130(5):774–84.

7. Arico' M, Scappaticci S, Danesio C. The genetics of Langerhans cell histiocytosis. In: Weitzman S, Egeler RM, editors. Histiocytic disorders of children and adults. Cambridge (United Kingdom): Cambridge University Press; 2005. p. 83–94.
8. Ribeiro KB, Degar B, Antoneli CBG, et al. Ethnicity, race, and socioeconomic status influence incidence of Langerhans cell histiocytosis. Pediatr Blood Cancer 2015;62(6):982–7.
9. Venkatramani R, Rosenberg S, Indramohan G, et al. An exploratory epidemiological study of Langerhans cell histiocytosis. Pediatr Blood Cancer 2012;59(7): 1324–6.
10. Hamre M, Hedberg J, Buckley J, et al. Langerhans cell histiocytosis: an exploratory epidemiologic study of 177 cases. Med Pediatr Oncol 1997;28(2):92–7.
11. Akefeldt SO, Finnstrom O, Gavhed D, et al. Langerhans cell histiocytosis in children born 1982-2005 after in vitro fertilization. Acta Paediatr 2012;101(11):1151–5.
12. Abla O, Egeler RM, Weitzman S. Langerhans cell histiocytosis: current concepts and treatments. Cancer Treat Rev 2010;36(4):354–9.
13. Hyman DM, Diamond EL, Vibat CRT, et al. Prospective blinded study of BRAFV600E mutation detection in cell-free DNA of patients with systemic histiocytic disorders. Cancer Discov 2015;5(1):64–71.
14. Howarth D, Gilchrist G, Mullan B, et al. Langerhans cell histiocytosis: diagnosis, natural history, management, and outcome. Cancer 1999;85:2278–90.
15. Donadieu J, Egeler RM, Pritchard J. Langerhans cell histiocytosis: a clinical update. In: Weitzman S, Egeler RM, editors. Histiocytic disorders of children and adults. Cambridge (United Kingdom): Cambridge University Press; 2005. p. 95–129.
16. Kilpatrick SE, Wenger DE, Gilchrist GS, et al. Langerhans' cell histiocytosis (histiocytosis X) of bone. A clinicopathologic analysis of 263 pediatric and adult cases. Cancer 1995;76(12):2471–84.
17. Lau L, Krafchik B, Trebo MM, et al. Cutaneous Langerhans cell histiocytosis in children under one year. Pediatr Blood Cancer 2006;46(1):66–71.
18. Grois N, Fahrner B, Arceci RJ, et al. Central nervous system disease in Langerhans cell histiocytosis. J Pediatr 2010;156(6):873–81, 881.e1.
19. Tazi A. Adult pulmonary Langerhans' cell histiocytosis. Eur Respir J 2006;27(6): 1272–85.
20. Galluzzo ML, Braier J, Rosenzweig SD, et al. Bone marrow findings at diagnosis in patients with multisystem Langerhans cell histiocytosis. Pediatr Developmental Pathol 2010;13(2):101–6.
21. Lahey ME. Histiocytosis X: an analysis of prognostic factors. J Pediatr 1975;87: 184–9.
22. Komp DM, Herson J, Starling KA, et al. A staging system for histiocytosis X: a Southwest Oncology Group study. Cancer 1981;47(4):798–800.
23. Gadner H, Grois N, Arico M, et al. A randomized trial of treatment for multisystem Langerhans' cell histiocytosis. J Pediatr 2001;138:728–34.
24. Minkov M, Grois N, Heitger A, et al. Response to initial treatment of multisystem Langerhans cell histiocytosis: an important prognostic indicator. Med Pediatr Oncol 2002;39(6):581–5.
25. Gadner H, Grois N, P"tschger U, et al. Improved outcome in multisystem Langerhans cell histiocytosis is associated with therapy intensification. Blood 2008; 111(5):2556–62.
26. Gadner H, Minkov M, Grois N, et al. Therapy prolongation improves outcome in multisystem Langerhans cell histiocytosis. Blood 2013;121(25):5006–14.

27. Ronceray L, Potschger U, Janka G, et al, German Society for Pediatric Hematology and Oncology. Pulmonary involvement in pediatric-onset multisystem Langerhans cell histiocytosis: effect on course and outcome. J Pediatr 2012;161(1): 129–33.e1–3.

28. Gadner H, Heitger A, Grois N, et al. Treatment strategy for disseminated Langerhans cell histiocytosis. DAL HX-83 Study Group. Med Pediatr Oncol 1994;23(2): 72–80.

29. Minkov M, Grois N, Heitger A, et al. Treatment of multisystem Langerhans cell histiocytosis. Results of the DAL-HX 83 and DAL-HX 90 studies. Klin Padiatr 2000;212(04):139–44.

30. Morimoto A, Ikushima S, Kinugawa N, et al. Improved outcome in the treatment of pediatric multifocal Langerhans cell histiocytosis: results from the Japan Langerhans Cell Histiocytosis Study Group-96 protocol study. Cancer 2006;107(3): 613–9.

31. Egeler RM, de Kraker J, Voûte PA. Cytosine-arabinoside, vincristine, and prednisolone in the treatment of children with disseminated Langerhans cell histiocytosis with organ dysfunction: experience at a single institution. Med Pediatr Oncol 1993;21(4):265–70.

32. Simko SJ, McClain KL, Allen CE. Up-front therapy for LCH: is it time to test an alternative to vinblastine/prednisone? Br J Haematol 2015;169(2):299–301.

33. Imashuku S, Kinugawa N, Matsuzaki A, et al. Langerhans cell histiocytosis with multifocal bone lesions: comparative clinical features between single and multisystems. Int J Hematol 2009;90(4):506–12.

34. Womer RB, Anunciato KR, Chehrenama M. Oral methotrexate and alternate-day prednisone for low-risk Langerhans cell histiocytosis. Med Pediatr Oncol 1995; 25:70–3.

35. Munn SE, Olliver L, Broadbent V, et al. Use of indomethacin in Langerhans cell histiocytosis. Med Pediatr Oncol 1999;32(4):247–9.

36. Braier J, Rosso D, Pollono D, et al. Symptomatic bone Langerhans cell histiocytosis treated at diagnosis or after reactivation with indomethacin alone. J Pediatr Hematol Oncol 2014;36:280–4.

37. Morimoto A, Shioda Y, Imamura T, et al. Nationwide survey of bisphosphonate therapy for children with reactivated Langerhans cell histiocytosis in Japan. Pediatr Blood Cancer 2011;56(1):110–5.

38. Haroche J, Cohen-Aubart F, Emile JF, et al. Dramatic efficacy of vemurafenib in both multisystemic and refractory Erdheim-Chester disease and Langerhans cell histiocytosis harboring the BRAF V600E mutation. Blood 2013;121(9): 1495–500.

39. Rodriguez-Galindo C, Kelly P, Jeng M, et al. Treatment of children with Langerhans cell histiocytosis with 2-chlorodeoxyadenosine. Am J Hematol 2002;69(3): 179–84.

40. Abraham A, Alsultan A, Jeng M, et al. Clofarabine salvage therapy for refractory high-risk Langerhans cell histiocytosis. Pediatr Blood Cancer 2013;60(6):E19–22.

41. Simko SJ, Tran HD, Jones J, et al. Clofarabine salvage therapy in refractory multifocal histiocytic disorders, including Langerhans cell histiocytosis, juvenile xanthogranuloma and Rosai–Dorfman disease. Pediatr Blood Cancer 2014; 61(3):479–87.

42. Bernard F, Thomas C, Bertrand Y, et al. Multicentre pilot study of 2-chlorodeoxyadenosine and cytosine arabinoside combined chemotherapy in refractory Langerhans cell histiocytosis with hematological dysfunction. Eur J Cancer 2005; 41(17):2682–9.

43. Steiner M, Mathes-Martin S, Attarbaschi A, et al. Improved outcome of treatment-resistant high-risk Langerhans cell histiocytosis after allogeneic stem cell transplantation with reduced-intensity conditioning. Bone Marrow Transpl 2005; 36(3):215–25.

44. Santana VM, Mirro J, Kearns C, et al. 2-chlorodeoxyadenosine produces a high rate of complete hematologic remission in relapsed acute myeloid leukemia. J Clin Oncol 1992;10:364–70.

45. Saven A, Burian C. Cladribine activity in adult Langerhans-cell histiocytosis. Blood 1999;93(12):4125–30.

46. Mottl H, Stary J, Chanova M, et al. Treatment of recurrent Langerhans cell histiocytosis in children with 2-chlorodeoxyadenosine. Leuk Lymphoma 2006;47(9): 1881–4.

47. Weitzman S, Wayne AS, Arceci R, et al. Nucleoside analogues in the therapy of Langerhans cell histiocytosis: a survey of members of the Histiocyte Society and review of the literature. Med Pediatr Oncol 1999;33:476–81.

48. Stine KC, Saylors RL, Saccente S, et al. Efficacy of continuous infusion 2-CDA (cladribine) in pediatric patients with Langerhans cell histiocytosis. Pediatr Blood Cancer 2004;43(1):81–4.

49. Dhall G, Finlay JL, Dunkel IJ, et al. Analysis of outcome for patients with mass lesions of the central nervous system due to Langerhans cell histiocytosis treated with 2-chlorodeoxyadenosine. Pediatr Blood Cancer 2008;50(1):72–9.

50. Choi EK, Park SR, Lee JH, et al. Induction of apoptosis by carboplatin and hyperthermia alone or combined in WERI human retinoblastoma cells. Int J Hyperthermia 2003;19(4):431–43.

51. Rosso DA, Amaral D, Latella A, et al. Reduced doses of cladribine and cytarabine regimen was effective and well tolerated in patients with refractory-risk multisystem Langerhans cell histiocytosis. Br J Haematol 2015. [Epub ahead of print].

52. Jeha S, Kantarjian H. Clofarabine for the treatment of acute lymphoblastic leukemia. Expert Rev Anticancer Ther 2007;7(2):113–8.

53. Moore AS, Kearns PR, Knapper S, et al. Novel therapies for children with acute myeloid leukaemia. Leukemia 2013;27(7):1451–60.

54. Rodriguez-Galindo C, Jeng M, Khuu P, et al. Clofarabine in refractory Langerhans cell histiocytosis. Pediatr Blood Cancer 2008;51(5):703–6.

55. Allen CE, Flores R, Rauch R, et al. Neurodegenerative central nervous system Langerhans cell histiocytosis and coincident hydrocephalus treated with vincristine/cytosine arabinoside. Pediatr Blood Cancer 2010;54(3):416–23.

56. Tsuda H, Yamasaki H, Tsuji T. Resolution of bone lysis in Langerhans cell histiocytosis by bisphosphonate therapy. Br J Haematol 2011;154(3):287.

57. Sivendran S, Harvey H, Lipton A, et al. Treatment of Langerhans cell histiocytosis bone lesions with zoledronic acid: a case series. Int J Hematol 2011;93(6):782–6.

58. Berres ML, Lim KP, Peters T, et al. BRAF-V600E expression in precursor versus differentiated dendritic cells defines clinically distinct LCH risk groups. J Exp Med 2014;211(4):669–83.

59. Haroche J, Charlotte F, Arnaud L, et al. High prevalence of BRAF V600E mutations in Erdheim-Chester disease but not in other non-Langerhans cell histiocytoses. Blood 2012;120(13):2700–3.

60. Haroche J, Cohen-Aubart F, Emile JF, et al. Reproducible and sustained efficacy of targeted therapy with vemurafenib in patients with BRAF(V600E)-mutated Erdheim-Chester disease. J Clin Oncol 2015;33(5):411–8.

61. Janku F, Amin HM, Yang D, et al. Response of histiocytoses to imatinib mesylate: fire to ashes. J Clin Oncol 2010;28(31):e633–6.

62. Kudo K, Ohga S, Morimoto A, et al. Improved outcome of refractory Langerhans cell histiocytosis in children with hematopoietic stem cell transplantation in Japan. Bone Marrow Transpl 2010;45(5):901–6.
63. Girschikofsky M, Arico M, Castillo D, et al. Management of adult patients with Langerhans cell histiocytosis: recommendations from an expert panel on behalf of Euro-Histio-Net. Orphanet J Rare Dis 2013;8:72.
64. Pierro J, Vaiselbuh SR. Adult Langerhans cell histiocytosis as a diagnostic pitfall. J Clin Oncol 2014. [Epub ahead of print].
65. Arico M, Girschikofsky M, Genereau T, et al. Langerhans cell histiocytosis in adults. Report from the international registry of the Histiocyte Society. Eur J Cancer 2003;39:2341–8.
66. Arico' M, Juli ED, Genereau T, et al. Special aspects of Langerhans cell histiocytosis in adult. In: Weitzman S, Egeler RM, editors. Histiocytic disorders of children and adults. Cambridge (United Kingdom): Cambridge University Press; 2005. p. 174–86.
67. Imafuku S, Shibata S, Tashiro A, et al. Cutaneous Langerhans cell histiocytosis in an elderly man successfully treated with narrowband ultraviolet B. Br J Dermatol 2007;157(6):1277–9.
68. Steen AE, Steen KH, Bauer R, et al. Successful treatment of cutaneous Langerhans cell histiocytosis with low-dose methotrexate. Br J Dermatol 2001;145(1): 137–40.
69. Minami M, Shima T, Kato K, et al. Successful treatment of adult Langerhans cell histiocytosis with intensified chemotherapy. Int J Hematol 2015. [Epub ahead of print].
70. Roden AC, Hu X, Kip S, et al. BRAF V600E expression in Langerhans cell histiocytosis: clinical and immunohistochemical study on 25 pulmonary and 54 extrapulmonary cases. Am J Surg Pathol 2014;38(4):548–51.
71. Lorillon G, Bergeron A, Detourmignies L, et al. Cladribine is effective against cystic pulmonary Langerhans cell histiocytosis. Am J Respir Crit Care Med 2012;186(9):930–2.
72. Dauriat G, Mal H, Thabut G, et al. Lung transplantation for pulmonary Langerhans' cell histiocytosis: a multicenter analysis. Transplantation 2006;81(5): 746–50.
73. Haupt R, Minkov M, Astigarraga I, et al. Langerhans cell histiocytosis (LCH): guidelines for diagnosis, clinical work-up, and treatment for patients till the age of 18 years. Pediatr Blood Cancer 2013;60(2):175–84.
74. Haupt R, Nanduri V, Calevo MG, et al. Permanent consequences in Langerhans cell histiocytosis patients: a pilot study from the Histiocyte Society-Late Effects Study Group. Pediatr Blood Cancer 2004;42(5):438–44.
75. Donadieu J, Rolon M-A, Thomas C, et al. Endocrine involvement in pediatric-onset Langerhans' cell histiocytosis: a population-based study. J Pediatr 2004; 144(3):344–50.
76. Donadieu J, Rolon M-A, Pion I, et al. Incidence of growth hormone deficiency in pediatric-onset Langerhans cell histiocytosis: efficacy and safety of growth hormone treatment. J Clin Endocrinol Metab 2004;89(2):604–9.
77. Prosch H, Grois N, Wnorowski M, et al. Long-term MR imaging course of neuro-degenerative Langerhans cell histiocytosis. AJNR Am J Neuroradiol 2007;28(6): 1022–8.
78. Ng Wing Tin S, Martin-Duverneuil N, Idbaih A, et al. Efficacy of vinblastine in central nervous system Langerhans cell histiocytosis: a nationwide retrospective study. Orphanet J Rare Dis 2011;6(1):83.

79. Imashuku S, Shioda Y, Kobayashi R, et al. Neurodegenerative central nervous system disease as late sequelae of Langerhans cell histiocytosis. Report from the Japan LCH Study Group. Haematologica 2008;93:615–8.
80. Chohan G, Barnett Y, Gibson J, et al. Langerhans cell histiocytosis with refractory central nervous system involvement responsive to infliximab. J Neurol Neurosurg Psychiatry 2012;83(5):573–5.
81. Idbaih A, Donadieu J, Barthez M, et al. Retinoic acid therapy in "degenerative-like" neuro-Langerhans cell histiocytosis: a prospective pilot study. Pediatr Blood Cancer 2004;43:55–8.

Strategies for the Prevention of Central Nervous System Complications in Patients with Langerhans Cell Histiocytosis

The Problem of Neurodegenerative Syndrome

Shinsaku Imashuku, MD, PhD[a],*, Robert J. Arceci, MD, PhD[b],†

KEYWORDS

- Langerhans cell histiocytosis • Central nervous system • Diabetes insipidus
- Neurodegenerative disease • Neuroinflammatory disease

KEY POINTS

- The syndrome of neurodegeneration-central nervous system-Langerhans cell histiocytosis (ND-CNS-LCH) in a subset of patients with LCH remains a progressive and devastating complication. Although a definitive incidence of this clinical syndrome remains unclear, estimates suggest around 10%. Patients at high risk for developing ND-CNS-LCH usually have disease involvement of the mastoid, temporal, and orbital bones as well as having developed diabetes insipidus.

- ND-CNS-LCH is usually a waxing and waning, yet progressive, disorder characterized by radiographic involvement of the cerebellar peduncles, basal ganglia, and often pons. Clinical signs and symptoms include problems with physical coordination (ataxia, dysarthria, dysmetria) as well as neurocognitive and psychological difficulties.

- The cause of ND-CNS-LCH is unknown, but seems to be in part mediated by CD8-positive lymphocytes and neuroinflammatory cytokines/chemokines. Whether ND-CNS-LCH is due to the presence of active, yet undetectable by current methods, LCH, or a paraneoplastic consequence of dendritic cell activation of the immune system to recognize CNS antigens is unknown.

- Several attempts at treatment with immunosuppressive or cytotoxic/immunosuppressive approaches have not resulted in an optimal strategy. There is a great need for prospective, randomized trials that will also measure critical biological and clinical characteristics of patients with new onset ND-CNS-LCH as well as for newly diagnosed patients with LCH at high risk for developing ND-CNS-LCH.

[a] Division of Hematology, Takasago-Seibu Hospital, 1-10-41 Nakasuji, Takasago 676-0812, Japan;
[b] Children's Center for Cancer and Blood Disorders, Department of Child Health, Phoenix Children's Hospital, University of Arizona College of Medicine, 445 North 5th Street, Suite 322, Phoenix, AZ 85004, USA
† Deceased.
* Corresponding author.
E-mail address: shinim95@mbox.kyoto-inet.or.jp

Hematol Oncol Clin N Am 29 (2015) 875–893
http://dx.doi.org/10.1016/j.hoc.2015.06.006
0889-8588/15/$ – see front matter © 2015 Elsevier Inc. All rights reserved.

hemonc.theclinics.com

INTRODUCTION

Langerhans cell histiocytosis (LCH) is a myeloid precursor/dendritic-cell-related histiocytosis; approximately two-thirds of those affected are children.[1] LCH is characterized by mutations of genes of the ERK signaling pathway as well as a lesional "cytokine storm," a term referring to both the high level and the diversity of locally synthesized cytokines.[2–10] Thus, in many ways and like many other neoplastic disorders, LCH can be considered an inflammatory neoplasia, meaning that although proliferation and survival of the neoplastic cells are driven by key genetic changes, the pathophysiology of the neoplasia is modified by the interchange of the neoplastic cells with their microenvironment and vice versa. Thus, increased levels of several of a variety of cytokines/chemokines have been found in the plasma/serum of patients with active LCH, and these levels typically reflect systemic disease activity (**Table 1**).[11,12]

Central nervous system (CNS) lesions are also common in LCH. These lesions include active lesions (ie, clear involvement with lesional LCH cells) involving the hypothalamic-pituitary axis with secondary central diabetes insipidus (CDI), space-occupying lesions at other sites, and neurodegenerative (ND) lesions of the cerebellum and basal ganglia.[13,14] Patients with an increased risk for the development of CNS lesions have been defined among patients with LCH.[15,16] Besides permanent CDI, the development of ND-CNS-LCH represents the most serious late CNS sequela.[13,17–19]

One of the hypotheses regarding CNS neurodegenerative disease (NDD) is that the level of CNS lesional cytokines/chemokines at disease onset may contribute to the subsequent development of CDI and ND-CNS-LCH disease, and that this level will be reflected in the cerebrospinal fluid (CSF). This hypothesis is based on consideration of relevant studies on serum/plasma measurements reflecting systemic disease activity. To date, there are reports concerning cytologic findings in CNS-LCH[17,20];

Table 1
Cytokines/chemokines as biomarkers in patients with Langerhans cell histiocytosis

Investigated Biological Materials	Cytokines/Chemokines Involved	References
Lesional	IL-1, IL-6, M-CSF[2], GM-CSF[2], TNFα, IL-3, CD40L, RANKL-RANL CCR6-CCL20, CCR7, CCL5, CXCR3-CXCL11	7–10
Systemic (serum/plasma)	IL-1RA, TNFα, IL-1β, CD40L, RANK, RANKL, OPG, sIL-2R	11,12
CSF[1] (cerebrospinal fluid)	In active CNS disease: Presence of CD1a positive cells	20
	In cases of ND-CNS-LCH: Increased NFL, GFAP, TAU	21
	Other biomarkers at the onset of active disease in patients at high risk for CNS-LCH: IL-6, TNFα, IL-8, Opn, DcR3, sCD27, MMP-9, MMP-9/TIMP-1 ratio, RANKL-RANL, OPG, CXCL10, CXCL 11, CXCL 13, others	Needs to be studied

Abbreviations: CCL, CC chemokine ligand; CCR, CC chemokine receptor; CSF[2], colony-stimulating factor; CXCR, CXC chemokine receptor; CXCL, CXC chemokine ligand; DcR3, decoy receptor 3; GFAp, glial fibrillary acid protein; NFL, neurofilament protein light chain; OPG, osteoprotegerin; Opn, osteopontin; RANK, receptor activator of NF-κB; RANKL, RANK ligand; MMP, matrix metalloproteinase; TAU, total τ protein, ligand; TIMP, tissue inhibitor of metalloproteinases.
   Data from Refs.[7–12,20,21]

however, only one CSF study has been performed to determine cytokines/chemo-kines activity within the CNS in patients with ND-CNS-LCH.[21]

The paucity of such data for patients with LCH, in contrast to leukemia and lymphoma, is in part due to the fact that lumbar puncture is not a routine procedure in the management of LCH. Thus, lumbar punctures would need to be considered as research studies at this time for patients with LCH, and this has not routinely been incorporated into prospective trials for these patients.[22] The determination of such cytokine/chemokine profiles as well as determination of the cell types, gene mutation determination, and proteomic analysis at the time of diagnosis in at least all high-risk patients would be potentially worthwhile to identify possible predictive biomarkers at disease onset and at times of reactivation as well as when CNS NDD radiographic or clinical findings are noted.

Inflammatory processes commonly play an important role in the pathway that leads to neuronal cell death in many NDDs (**Fig. 1**). The inflammatory response usually involves the perivascular area. Here, invading T cells interact with the activated microglia, which are resident immune cells of the CNS and serve as a pathologic hallmark of inflammatory brain disease. Chronic activation of the microglia may result in neuronal damage because of the release of cytotoxic molecules, such as proinflammatory cytokines, reactive oxygen intermediates, proteinases, and complement proteins.[23] The suppression of microglia-mediated inflammation may thus represent an important prophylactic or therapeutic strategy for the management of ND-CNS-LCH disease. The facilitation of neuroprotection may also be important, such as through the use of agents that target the trafficking of blood cells into the CNS.

This review presents data on findings regarding LCH-related CNS findings, including the CSF profiles of cytokines/chemokines and other molecular factors in a range of neurologic diseases. Second, it discusses which CSF analyses may be indicated for study in patients with LCH, and the development of clinical trials to test strategies for the prevention of CNS-LCH lesions. The overall goal is to demonstrate a conceptual framework in which to further develop optimal therapeutic strategies for patients at high risk for the development of CNS-LCH.

LABORATORY STUDIES OF RELEVANCE TO CENTRAL NERVOUS SYSTEM-LANGERHANS CELL HISTIOCYTOSIS DISEASE
Cytokines/Chemokines and Other Cerebrospinal Fluid Markers in Neuroinflammatory Diseases

Most of the cytokines/chemokines that have been tested in the CSF of patients with neuroinflammatory disease have been proinflammatory cytokines (interleukin [IL]-1β, IL-6, and IL-8) and chemokines associated with Th1 CXC chemokine ligand (CXCL9-11), Th2 (CCL22), and B cells (CXCL13) (see **Table 1**). Chemokines and their receptors are involved in T-cell trafficking into the CNS.[24,25] In particular, the chemokine CXCL10 regulates the migration of activated T cells into the CNS by binding to the CXC chemokine receptor (CXCR3).[24] Increased levels of CCL5, CXCL10, CXCL12, and CCL19 in the CSF of patients with neuroinflammation have been reported.[26] Osteopontin (Opn), a cytokine with a pivotal role in cellular immune responses, has been found to be elevated in the CSF of patients with a variety of neuroinflammatory diseases.[27–29] In contrast, although high CSF concentrations of the decoy receptor 3 (DcR3) have been found in a range of neurologic diseases, it was barely detectable in the serum of affected patients.[30] DcR3 is a member of the TNF receptor superfamily and was initially thought to inhibit the cytokine responses of FasL. DcR3 has also been shown to induce the formation of osteoclasts from human monocytes.[31]

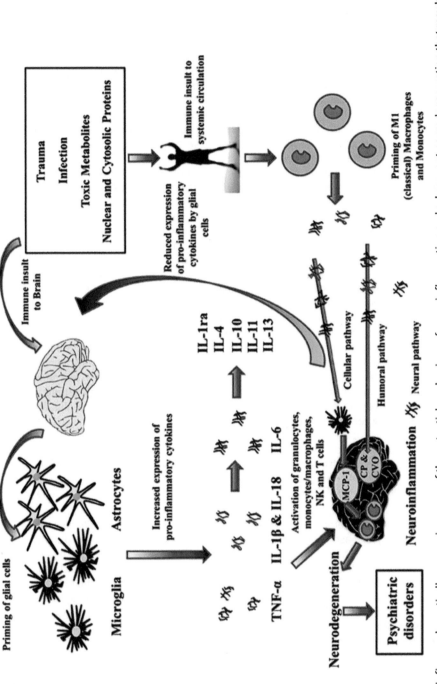

Fig. 1. This figure schematically summarizes some of the potential mechanisms of neuroinflammation and subsequent neurodegeneration that may be related to psychiatric disorders. Such mechanisms of neuroinflammation are likely to play important roles in other disorders, such as ND-CNS-LCH, characterized by neuroinflammatory and neurodegeneration. Importantly, many of these mechanisms demonstrate interactions between the CNS and systemic changes. CP, choroid plexus; CVO, circumventricular organs; MCP-1, monocyte chemoattractant protein-1; NK, natural killer. (*From* Singhal G, Jaehne EJ, Corrigan F, et al. Inflammasomes in neuroinflammation and changes in brain function: a focused review. Front Neurosci 2014;8:315; with permission.)

High CSF levels of IL-6, IL-12, IL-1β, and tumor necrosis factor-α (TNF-α) distinguish bacterial from aseptic meningitis.[32–34] IL-6, IL-8, and TNF-α in CSF are particularly important mediators of the meningeal inflammatory process.[35] Increased CSF concentrations of TNF-α, IL-1-α, and IL-6 have also been reported in pediatric patients with acute encephalitis/encephalopathy.[36] Increased CSF levels of TNF-α, IL-1ra, and CXCL8 have been demonstrated in patients with malaria.[37,38] In patients with tick-borne encephalitis, the detection of increased CSF concentration of CXCL10 suggests that this chemokine may play a role in the recruitment of CXCR3-expressing T cells into the CNS.[39] Increased CSF levels of CXCL10 in subacute sclerosing panencephalitis, and of CXCL11 in acute neuroborreliosis, have also been reported.[25,40] High CSF levels of Opn have been reported in patients with HIV-associated dementia.[28]

In patients with multiple sclerosis (MS), elevated IL-1β in CSF is a predictive biomarker for active disease.[41] Significantly increased CSF concentrations of CXCL10 have also been reported, whereas the CSF concentrations of CCL2 were found to be reduced in MS, compared with those in control groups.[42] The levels of CXCL8 and CCL2 were found to be higher in CFS than in serum, and significantly increased levels of CXCL8 and CCL5 were observed during relapse.[43] In MS, it has been hypothesized that CXCL13 plays a major role in the CNS recruitment of B cells and T cells that express the chemokine receptor CXCR5; these molecules are thus potential therapeutic targets.[44] Mellergård and colleagues[45] demonstrated a decrease in the CSF concentration of CXCL13 in patients with MS who had received high-dose methylprednisolone and natalizumab. High CSF concentrations of Opn have also been reported in MS.[27,29]

Increased CSF levels of CCL2 and CXCL10 have been reported in Guillain-Barre syndrome, and increased levels of macrophage inflammatory protein-3 beta (MIP-3β) and interferon gamma inducible protein 10 (IP-10) have been reported in chronic inflammatory demyelinating polyradiculoneuropathy.[46] DcR3 has been shown to be a potential suppressor of experimental autoimmune encephalitis in experiments involving its intrathecal administration in mice.[47] In one patient with neuro-Sweet disease, CSF concentrations of IL-6, interferon-γ (IFN-γ), CXCL8, and CXCL10 were found to be substantially higher than in control subjects with other neurologic diseases.[48] Increased CSF levels of IL-6 have also been reported in neuro-Behçet syndrome.[49]

Most NDDs of the CNS are associated with microglia-mediated inflammation, and CD40 signaling plays a critical role in this process.[50] Increased activation of the CD40-CD40L complex is found in major forms of dementia, and this leads to the increased synthesis of proinflammatory cytokines by immune cells in the CNS.[51] Of interest, similarly high serum concentrations of soluble CD40L (sCD154) have been demonstrated in patients with multifocal LCH.[11] Measurement of the concentration of soluble CD40L (sCD154) in CSF may thus be worthwhile to investigate in patients with LCH.

Increased soluble TNF is a hallmark of acute and chronic neuroinflammation as well as of many NDDs.[52] The CSF concentrations of MCP-1 and IL-8 were found to be significantly higher in patients with amyotrophic lateral sclerosis than in controls.[53] In postpolio syndrome (PPS), high CSF levels of IFN-γ, TNF-α mRNA, IL-2, and sIL-2R have been reported.[54,55]

In multiple myeloma (MM), DcR3 is synthesized by myeloma cells and then interacts with FasL, a process that has been found to inhibit osteoclast apoptosis,[56] which may, in turn, contribute to the osteolytic aspect of myeloma. However, the level of DcR3 in the CSF has not yet been established in MM. In patients with CNS lymphoma, Fischer and colleagues[57] assessed levels of CXCL12 and CXCL13 in both CSF and serum and found that the CSF concentration of CXCL13 was correlated with the degree of blood-brain barrier (BBB) disruption. Patients with CNS lymphoma have also been shown to have high CSF concentrations of soluble CD27/DPP4 (dipeptidyl peptidase-4), an enzyme with known immunostimulating activity.[58]

Matrix Metalloproteinases and Other Cerebrospinal Fluid Molecules in Neuroinflammatory Diseases

Extracellular matrix glycoproteins are components of cell-cell boundaries within the microvascular and extravascular tissues of the CNS. Matrix metalloproteinases (MMPs) are involved in the migration of leukocytes into the CNS during inflammation.[59] Release of MMPs into the CSF may indicate CNS inflammatory disease or disruption of the BBB following an ischemic cerebrovascular accident.[60] Activated microglia are known to secrete MMP.[61] Soluble forms of vascular cell adhesion molecule-1, intracellular adhesion molecule-1 (ICAM-1), and E-Selectin play key roles in the response to BBB injury and are considered biomarkers of disease activity in MS.[62] The CSF concentrations of the nerve/glial cell marker proteins, such as glial fibrillary acidic protein (GFAP), light subunit of neurofilament protein (NFL), and neuron-specific enolase (NSE), have been assayed in various neuroinjury and ND disorders (**Table 2**).[63,64] In Lyme neuroborreliosis with meningoradiculitis, the pretreatment CSF levels of GFAP and NFL were correlated with clinical outcome, and they declined significantly in response to treatment.[63]

Increased CSF levels of MMP-9 have been reported in viral, bacterial, and fungal meningitis; the concentrations of tissue inhibitor of metalloproteinases (TIMP-1) were found to greatly exceed those of MMP-9.[65–68] MMPs are thought to be involved in demyelination and the disruption of the BBB in MS. MMP-9, in particular, is considered a marker of MS pathogenesis. Active MMP-9 and the MMP-9/TIMP-1 ratio have been found to be increased in the CSF of patients with MS.[59] The MMP-9/TIMP-1 ratio was also found to be significantly increased in neuro-Behçet disease, and polymorphonuclear cells were identified as one source of the MMP-9 that was detected in the CSF.[69] Because the serum concentrations of MMP and TIMP-1 are much higher than those in the CSF, it has been hypothesized that the serum active MMP-9/TIMP-1 ratio may be a useful surrogate marker for the monitoring of neuroinflammatory disease activity.[59] Mitosek-Szewczyk and colleagues[62] showed reduction of concentrations of soluble intercellular adhesion molecule-1 (sICAM-1) and sE-Selectin in serum, but not in CSF, after cladribine therapy in patients with remitting-relapsing MS.

The NSE level in CSF is of prognostic value in acute cerebellar ataxia.[70] High CSF levels of NSE, GFAP, and NFL have been reported in patients with acute lymphocytic leukemia, and it has been suggested that these increases can be interpreted as early signs of brain injury.[64] Gonzalez and colleagues[71] performed proteomic profile studies in PPS and identified novel candidate protein biomarkers. Other CSF biomarkers of neurodegeneration, carbonyl proteins,[72] and leucine-rich α2-glycoprotein[73] have been described. In ND-CNS-LCH, Gavhed and colleagues[21] reported increased levels of NFL, tau protein, and GFAP in a subset of their patient sample. Of these, the patients with most severe clinical and neuroradiological signs displayed the highest levels of NFL and GFAP.

Two types of NDD are due to an inborn error of metabolism.[74,75] One is brain iron accumulation, which is caused by mutations of the pantothenate kinase 2 (*PANK2*) gene,[75] and the other is infantile neuroaxonal dystrophy, which is caused by mutations in the gene encoding phospholipase A(2) group VI (*PLA2G6*).[74] No CSF studies have been reported for these diseases to date.

Autoantibodies and Neuroinflammation

The role of autoantibodies in the development of ND-CNS-LCH disease remains unknown. One report detected no autoantibodies to CNS tissue in patients with

Table 2
Cerebrospinal fluid cytokines/chemokines and other biomarkers identified in various neurologic diseases

Category	Disease	Increased Cytokines/Chemokines in CSF
CNS infections	Meningitis (bacterial, aseptic)	IL-6, IL-1β, IL-8, TNF-α, IL-12
	Encephalitis/encephalopathy	TNF-α, IL-1β, IL-6, IL-10, sTNFR1
	SSPE	IL-12, CXCL10
	Lyme neuroborreliosis	GFAP, NFL
Autoimmune diseases	Multiple sclerosis	IL-1Ra, IL-1RII
		CCL2, CCL5, CXCL10, CXCL8, DcR3 CXCL13
	Neuro-Sweet disease	IL-6, IFN-γ, CXCL8, CXCL10
	Neuro-Behçet disease	MMP-9, TIMP-1
NDDs	AD, PD	Tau-T, Aβ1-42, P-tau181P,
	ALS	MCP-1, IL-8
	PPS	IL-2, sIL-2R, mRNA of IFN-γ, TNFα
Autoantibody-related CNS disease	CDI, Sydenham chorea, encephalitis	AVPc-Abs, anti-basal ganglia-Abs, anti-NMDAR-Abs
Hemato-oncology	CNS lymphoma	CXCL13, sCD27, sIL-2R
	MM	DcR3
BBB disruption	Ischemia	MMP-9
Brain injury	ALL-related	NSE, GFAP, NFL, AsR
	Other	MBP, GFAP, NCAM, NSE
	Astrogial/neuronal interaction	GFAP, NFL

Abbreviations: ALL, acute lymphocytic leukemia; ALS, amyotrophic lateral sclerosis; anti-NMDAR-Abs, anti-*N*-methyl-D-aspartate receptor antibodies; AsR, ascorbyl radical; CCL, CC chemokine ligand; CCR, CC chemokine receptor; IL-1Ra, IL-1 receptor antagonist; MBP, myelin basic protein; MCP, monocyte chemotactic protein-1; NCAM, neural cell adhesion molecule; OPG, osteoprotegerin; RANK, Receptor activator of NF-κB; RANKL, RANK ligand; SSPE, subacute sclerosing panencephalitis; TAU, total τ protein, ligand; Tau-T, total tau.

ND-CNS-LCH.[76] However, there are some clear parallels between various paraneoplastic autoimmune syndromes that are due to antineuronal autoantibodies[77,78] and the paraneoplastic nature of ND-CNS-LCH. Autoantibodies have also been identified for CDI and for disorders of the basal ganglia. Maghnie and colleagues[79] reported the presence of circulating anti-vasopressin-cell antibodies (AVPc-Abs) in 9 patients with idiopathic CDI, 4 patients with LCH, and 2 patients with germinoma. Pivonello and colleagues[80] cautioned that AVPc-Abs may mask LCH or germinoma, and thus a diagnosis of CDI secondary to LCH must be assigned with caution. Antibasal ganglia antibodies have been detected in Sydenham chorea and other poststreptococcal neuropsychiatric disorders.[81,82] Anti-NMDAR (*N*-methyl-D-aspartate receptor) paraneoplastic encephalitis has been described and usually presents with disturbances of memory, behavior, and cognition.[83–85] Such findings suggest that studies are warranted to determine if autoantibodies of relevance to the development of ND-CNS-LCH disease can be observed in a consistent fashion in patients with new onset disease.

Complement Activation Cerebrospinal Fluid Markers in Neuroinflammatory and Neurodegenerative Diseases

CNS damage in neurologic disorders such as neuromyelitis optica (NMO) and myasthenia gravis has been shown to be in part mediated by the complement system.[86]

In these diseases, anti-APQ4 or anti-AChR autoantibodies can mediate complement-dependent cytotoxicity. Of various complement proteins (C3a, C4a, C5a, and sC5b-9) produced in complement activation, the C5a levels in CSF were elevated significantly and correlated with the severity of exacerbation in NMO patients.[87] Also, CSF levels of sC5b-9 are increased in patients with NMO, reflecting the activation of complement in the disease.[88] For such diseases, antibody-based C5 inhibitor eculizumab has been suggested to be of potential benefit as treatment.[89] In the pathogenesis of NDDs, the activation of the complement system was also proposed to be involved.[90] For instance, in Parkinson disease (PD), CSF levels of complement 3 and factor H were shown to predict the disease activity.[91]

Cerebrospinal Fluid Biomarkers in Alzheimer Disease and Parkinson Disease

Alzheimer disease (AD) and PD are the most common ND disorders.[92] In AD, extensive studies have been pursued to develop therapy that could slow or arrest disease progression.[93] CSF biomarkers have been extensively studied in AD and PD.[92–95] Particularly in AD, CSF biomarkers, such as total tau (tau-T), β-amyloid 1-42 (Aβ1-42), phosphorylated tau at threonine 181 (P-tau181P), are used in clinical practice in diagnosis and as markers for evaluating disease modification.[92,95,96] Investigators have found that abnormalities in CSF markers are associated with the development of mild cognitive impairment.[95] In PD, besides the above-mentioned markers, determination of NFL in CSF is said to be useful in the differential diagnosis between PD and other Parkinsonian syndromes.[94] These types of studies may help provide the basis for further investigation of CSF levels in LCH and early onset of ND-CNS-LCH.

LABORATORY AND THERAPEUTIC STUDIES TO PREVENT AND TREAT NEURODEGENERATION-CENTRAL NERVOUS SYSTEM-LANGERHANS CELL HISTIOCYTOSIS DISEASE

Patients at High Risk versus Low Risk for Central Nervous System-Langerhans Cell Histiocytosis

Patients with LCH lesions involving the temporal, petrous, orbital, and zygomatic bones have been found to be associated with a significantly higher incidence of CNS disease.[16,18] ND-CNS-LCH occurs most frequently in young patients presenting with skull/facial lesions at LCH disease onset.[13,19,76] It has therefore been hypothesized that the analysis of cytokines/chemokines and other CSF markers present at disease onset in patients at high risk for CNS disease will provide valuable insights into the pathogenesis of ND-CNS-LCH disease (see **Fig. 1**). These biomarkers may also facilitate the identification of patients who are at the highest risk for the development CNS disease.

Subclinical Versus Clinical Central Nervous System-Langerhans Cell Histiocytosis Lesions

Given that LCH is characterized by a lesional cytokine storm, high CSF concentrations of proinflammatory cytokines, such as IL-6 and TNF-α, may be expected in patients with clinically active ND-CNS-LCH disease as well as in those with subclinical disease identified by brain MRI scanning. High CSF concentrations of cytokines/chemokines at disease onset may also indicate the presence of MRI-negative microscopic CNS LCH lesions, which may herald the later onset of MRI-positive ND-CNS-LCH disease.

Thus, 2 key questions are whether a combination of CSF cytokine measurements and brain MRI at disease onset would (1) quantify the activity of clinical as well as subclinical lesions, and (2) predict the later development of CNS-LCH disease (**Fig. 2**). A further question is how soon CSF markers of neuroinjury and neurodegeneration

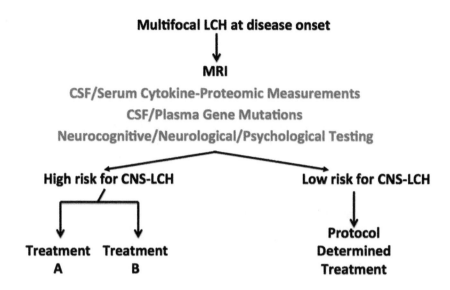

Fig. 2. Possible clinical model for testing novel agents with intent to reduce the chance of ND-CNS-LCH disease. Key elements include initial profiling to determine patients who are high risk for developing CNS-LCH (including pituitary involvement and NDD). Although currently used conventional risk factors can be used to stratify into 2 risk groups, additional testing, such as CSF/serum cytokine/chemokine measures, CSF/plasma gene mutation analysis, and practical neurocognitive/neurologic/psychological assessments, at the time of diagnosis and at set intervals during and after treatment according to 1 of 2 different treatments, such as chemotherapy plus or minus IVIG or 2 different chemotherapeutic regimens, might provide a basis for stratifying patients.

become detectable following the initial development of MRI-positive ND-CNS-LCH lesion.

Cerebrospinal Fluid Biomarkers and the Pathogenesis of Central Nervous System-Langerhans Cell Histiocytosis

CXCL10 and CXCL11 are 2 potential mediators that may play a role in the trafficking of T cells into the CNS in patients with ND-CNS-LCH. Opn is involved in cell-mediated and granulomatous inflammation.[97] Increased expression of Opn has been reported in CD207 (+) LCH cells[98] and high levels of Opn have been demonstrated in cells obtained by bronchopulmonary lavage from patients with pulmonary LCH.[99] The CSF concentration of Opn in patients with LCH may therefore be of particular interest to further study.

DcR3 seems to be one of the key cytokines in modulating Th17 immune responses and has been abundant in neuroinflammation in CSF.[30] Research suggests that DcR3 is a potential suppressor of CNS inflammation, and it has been proposed that this property is attributable to either the direct inhibition of CNS inflammation or the suppression of encephalitogenic Th17 cells.[47] IL-17A from Th17 cells[100] has been implicated in granuloma formation, neurodegeneration, and bone resorption. Intralesional expression of IL-17A has been detected in LCH tissue sections. In addition, high serum levels of IL-17A have been demonstrated in patients with active LCH,[101] although another study reported no evidence of IL-17A in LCH lesions or serum from affected patients.[102]

T-cell/microglia interactions may also be mediators of the CNS inflammatory response involving CNS-LCH lesions. The ingestion of apoptotic T cells by microglia is necessary for the efficient clearing of inflammatory infiltrates, which in turn can downregulate proinflammatory phagocyte immune functions in the CNS.[103,104] The persistence of the neuroinflammatory component of ND-CNS-LCH might be related to a defect in this process. It is possible that during the primary invasion of active LCH cells and other cells into the CNS, these immunomodulatory cells are not effectively removed. Measurement of CSF biomarkers of microglial activation, such as MMP-9, is, therefore, likely to be worthwhile, because the degree of microglial activation at disease onset might also be correlated with the development of ND-CNS-LCH. Furthermore, biomarkers used in the evaluation of patients with AD and PD may provide important clues for predicting the development or following patients with ND-CNS-LCH.

Determination of Cerebrospinal Fluid Cytokines/Chemokines Concentrations

A prediction for the evaluation of ND-CNS-LCH lesion-specific cytokines/chemokines is that their concentration in the CSF will be higher than that in plasma/sera. An important issue when assessing CSF concentrations of cytokines/chemokines is to also determine plasma/sera levels simultaneously. An aliquot of a cell suspension of CSF may also be submitted for flow cytometry, which can determine T-cell subsets as well as mRNA levels of cytokines/chemokines in CSF mononuclear cells.[53] Supernatants of each centrifuged CSF sample should also be saved safely in aliquots at $-70°C$ before the performance of assays for cytokines/chemokines as well as for testing for the presence of autoantibodies.[77–85] Importantly, this could also facilitate the exchange of material among different laboratories, thus increasing the possibility of meaningful numbers of patient samples through collaborative groups.

Treatment of Neurodegenerative-Central Nervous System-Langerhans Cell Histiocytosis

There is no established optimal therapy for patients who develop ND-CNS-LCH. In addition, as with other neuroinflammatory disorders that have a waxing and waning course, the assessment of response can be problematic. Such disorders can show stable signs and symptoms for prolonged periods of time and then progress rapidly only to again stabilize. The unlikely recovery of permanently damaged neurologic pathways does not provide the opportunity of observing reversal of clinical features. Acute or subacute episodes may provide unique windows on both understanding the pathophysiology and testing the potential efficacy of a therapeutic intervention. The rarity of the disease as well as a lack of conformity of assessing patients' signs and symptoms, radiographic findings, and criteria for response to interventions further complicates conclusions that can be made. Several approaches, including the use of immunosuppressive as well as cytotoxic-immunosuppressive agents, have nevertheless been tried.

Intravenous immune globulin (IVIG) has been used in the management of various autoimmune neurologic diseases, including ND-CNS-LCH. For example, IVIG has been shown to differentially modulate MMP-9 synthesis in resting and activated microglia in MS[59] and to reduce CSF cytokines in PPS.[54] IVIG has also been proposed as a potential immunotherapy agent for AD, because it contains anti-β-amyloid antibodies.[105,106] IVIG has been shown to be an effective therapeutic agent for Sydenham chorea, a disease in which antibasal ganglia antibodies are implicated.[107] The use of IVIG in patients with ND-CNS-LCH has been reported to show improvement in signs and symptoms in some patients.[22,108–110] In these studies, IVIG alone or in combination with chemotherapy regimens has been used, usually demonstrating stabilization of clinical features and occasionally with modest albeit transient improvements. All of these studies have involved very small numbers of patients in a nonrandomized or non-cross-over evaluation. There is a suggestion that early intervention when an Expanded Disability Status Scale score is low may be advantageous.[109]

Statins also have anti-inflammatory and immunomodulatory properties, in part through their suppression of CD40 signaling, which is involved in microglial immune responses in the CNS.[50] TNF is an attractive therapeutic target for the treatment of acute and chronic NDDs. Positive responses to infliximab have been reported in neurosarcoidosis.[111,112] However, a major limitation of the anti-TNF-α agents, such as infliximab and etanercept, is that they have a limited capacity to cross the BBB. Thalidomide and its analogues have been proposed for the treatment of ND-CNS-LCH because of their anti-TNF-α activity,[113] but have not been carefully tested. The use of high doses of steroids has also not proven to be terribly useful, but again has not been studied in detail.[14]

Cytotoxic-immunosuppressive approaches have included several agents. Cladribine (2-chlorodeoxyadenosine or 2CDA) has both cytotoxic and immunosuppressive characteristics along with good CNS penetration. Cladribine has thus been used in patients with CNS LCH with demonstration of radiographic resolution of tumorous as well as typical brainstem ND-CNS-LCH changes on MRI; however, no definitive evidence that improvements in ND-CNS-LCH clinical features over time has been reported.[114–116] The use of low-dose cytarabine (100 mg/m^2 daily for 5 days) with or without vincristine has been reported in 8 patients, 4 of whom had complications from hydrocephalus; 3 patients developed stable disease with others showing eventual progression of symptoms.[117] All-trans retinoic acid was used to treat 10 patients with ND-CNS-LCH with no changes noted on follow-up MRIs; all patients reported to be clinically stable at 1 year.[118]

Opportunities for Prevention of Neurodegenerative-Central Nervous System-Langerhans Cell Histiocytosis

When available treatments for a devastating disease, such as ND-CNS-LCH, are suboptimal, the interventions designed to prevent that disease must take on an increasingly important role. However, major issues arise when considered how such studies should be done. For instance, the true incidence of ND-CNS-LCH with a contemporary standard therapy for patients with LCH would be needed in order to statistically power such a study adequately to achieve definitive conclusions. To this end, identifying a high-risk group and focusing the study on that group might make such a study more manageable and acceptable. Pretreatment and on-study assessments of neurologic, neuro-cognitive, and radiographic would need to be standardized, and, ideally, centrally reviewed. And as noted above, determination of presumed key biological CSF and serum biomarkers would be both timely and important. Another important question is to determine what treatment modalities should be studied, such as IVIG, a nucleoside inhibitor such as cladribine or clofarabine, cytarabine, or immunomodulators such as interleukin receptor (ILR) antagonists or B-cell-directed modalities like anti-CD20 monoclonal antibody to inhibit possible paraneoplastic-associated autoantibodies. The JLSG-96 and JLSG-02 studies reported that a combination of vincristine, cytarabine, and prednisolone did not result in prevention of ND-CNS-LCH. Based on data presented for IVIG as well as the use of cladribine in patients with

LCH and MS,[116,119–122] the Japanese cooperative group is considering testing the combination of IVIG plus cladribine as first-line chemotherapy.

An attempt to perform such a study is in progress with aims to (1) define a group of patients with highest risk of developing ND-CNS-LCH using CSF and serum analyses as well as other clinical features, and (2) to reduce or prevent ND-CNS-LCH using optimal therapeutic measures.

SUMMARY AND FUTURE DIRECTIONS

The development of the neurodegenerative syndrome associated with LCH remains a devastating complication without established standards of evaluation or treatment. However, there are many parallel features common to this disorder and several other neuroinflammatory/neurodegenerative disorders. A further important insight over the past several years has been recognition from both preclinical models and humans of the CNS consequences of severe systemic inflammatory conditions, including neurologic, neurocognitive, and psychologically adverse sequelae. This intimate association of body and brain is often driven by soluble immunomodulatory factors, such as, but not restricted to, cytokines and chemokines. These observations should be further examined in collaborative efforts with experts in those disciplines of autoimmune and paraneoplastic disorders.

Improved, evidence-based treatment of patients with ND-CNS-LCH is a glaring need. Because such definitive studies have not been yet accomplished by single institutions or small groups of collaborating institutions, it would seem imperative that consortia of sufficient size should focus their efforts on defining biological and clinical risk factors, standardizing practical and achievable quantitative assessments of neurologic, neurocognitive, and psychological deficits for baseline and subsequent on- and off-treatment monitoring, and muster the will to randomize treatment options, when possible, based on mechanistic data.

Another key area of importance is the need to define the features that characterize a group at highest risk of developing ND-CNS-LCH. Thus, first-line clinical trials need to include practical assessments of systemic and CNS biomarkers, including CSF and plasma testing for ERK pathway gene mutations, along with clinical and radiographic features with the intent of sharing those data possibly through controlled, crowd-sourcing platforms for integrative, predictive analysis. It is also possible that, while such a study is being done, currently defined groups with known higher risk for ND-CNS-LCH could be randomized based on evidence as it exists to different treatments that have both mechanistic and possibly some clinical evidence. Although preclinical evidence to support the development of clinical trials in LCH has not been previously possible, this may change with the generation of animal models designed to molecularly mimic the drivers of LCH in humans. Whether some of the agents that target mutated BRAF, MEK, or potentially other mutated proteins identified in LCH should be strongly considered for such trials.

REFERENCES

1. Weitzman S, Egeler RM. Histiocytic disorders of children and adults: introduction to the problem, overview, historical perspective and epidemiology. In: Weitzman S, Egeler RM, editors. Histiocytic discorders of children and adults. Cambridge (United Kingdom): Cambridge University Press; 2005. p. 1–13.
2. Badalian-Very G, Vergilio JA, Degar BA, et al. Recurrent BRAF mutations in Langerhans cell histiocytosis. Blood 2010;116(11):1919–23.

3. Badalian-Very G, Vergilio JA, Fleming M, et al. Pathogenesis of Langerhans cell histiocytosis. Annu Rev Pathol 2013;8:1–20.
4. Nelson DS, Quispel W, Badalian-Very G, et al. Somatic activating ARAF mutations in Langerhans cell histiocytosis. Blood 2014;123(20):3152–5.
5. Nelson DS, van Halteren A, Quispel WT, et al. MAP2K1 and MAP3K1 mutations in langerhans cell histiocytosis. Genes Chromosomes Cancer 2015;54(6): 361–8.
6. Chakraborty R, Hampton OA, Shen X, et al. Mutually exclusive recurrent somatic mutations in MAP2K1 and BRAF support a central role for ERK activation in LCH pathogenesis. Blood 2014;124(19):3007–15.
7. de Graaf JH, Tamminga RY, Kamps WA, et al. Langerhans' cell histiocytosis: expression of leukocyte cellular adhesion molecules suggests abnormal homing and differentiation. Am J Pathol 1994;144(3):466–72.
8. Egeler RM, Favara BE, van Meurs M, et al. Differential In situ cytokine profiles of Langerhans-like cells and T cells in Langerhans cell histiocytosis: abundant expression of cytokines relevant to disease and treatment. Blood 1999;94(12): 4195–201.
9. Annels NE, Da Costa CE, Prins FA, et al. Aberrant chemokine receptor expression and chemokine production by Langerhans cells underlies the pathogenesis of Langerhans cell histiocytosis. J Exp Med 2003;197(10):1385–90.
10. Beverley PC, Egeler RM, Arceci RJ, et al. The Nikolas Symposia and histiocytosis. Nat Rev Cancer 2005;5(6):488–94.
11. Ishii R, Morimoto A, Ikushima S, et al. High serum values of soluble CD154, IL-2 receptor, RANKL and osteoprotegerin in Langerhans cell histiocytosis. Pediatr Blood Cancer 2006;47(2):194–9.
12. Rosso DA, Ripoli MF, Roy A, et al. Serum levels of interleukin-1 receptor antagonist and tumor necrosis factor-alpha are elevated in children with Langerhans cell histiocytosis. J Pediatr Hematol Oncol 2003;25(6):480–3.
13. Grois N, Prayer D, Prosch H, et al, CNS LCH Co-operative Group. Neuropathology of CNS disease in Langerhans cell histiocytosis. Brain 2005;128(Pt 4): 829–38.
14. Grois NG, Favara BE, Mostbeck GH, et al. Central nervous system disease in Langerhans cell histiocytosis. Hematol Oncol Clin North Am 1998;12(2): 287–305.
15. Grois N, Potschger U, Prosch H, et al. Risk factors for diabetes insipidus in langerhans cell histiocytosis. Pediatr Blood Cancer 2006;46(2):228–33.
16. Imashuku S, Kinugawa N, Matsuzaki A, et al, Japan LCH Study Group. Langerhans cell histiocytosis with multifocal bone lesions: comparative clinical features between single and multi-systems. Int J Hematol 2009;90(4):506–12.
17. Ghosal N, Kapila K, Kakkar S, et al. Langerhans cell histiocytosis infiltration in cerebrospinal fluid: a case report. Diagn Cytopathol 2001;24(2):123–5.
18. Grois N, Posch H, Lassmann H, et al. Central nervous system disease in Langerhans cell histiocytosis. In: Weitzman S, Egeler RM, editors. Histiocytic disorders of children and adults. Cambridge (United Kingdom): Chambridge University Press; 2005. p. 208–28.
19. Imashuku S, Shioda Y, Kobayashi R, et al. Neurodegenerative central nervous system disease as late sequelae of Langerhans cell histiocytosis. Report from the Japan LCH Study Group. Haematologica 2008;93(4):615–8.
20. Prosch H, Feldges A, Grois N, et al. Demonstration of CD1a positive cells in the cerebrospinal fluid–a clue to diagnosis of isolated Langerhans cell histiocytosis of the hypothalamic-pituitary axis? Med Pediatr Oncol 2003;41(5):474–6.

21. Gavhed D, Akefeldt SO, Osterlundh G, et al. Biomarkers in the cerebrospinal fluid and neurodegeneration in Langerhans cell histiocytosis. Pediatr Blood Cancer 2009;53(7):1264–70.

22. Imashuku S. High dose immunoglobulin (IVIG) may reduce the incidence of Langerhans cell histiocytosis (LCH)-associated central nervous system involvement. CNS Neurol Disord Drug Targets 2009;8(5):380–6.

23. Dheen ST, Kaur C, Ling EA. Microglial activation and its implications in the brain diseases. Curr Med Chem 2007;14(11):1189–97.

24. Christensen JE, de Lemos C, Moos T, et al. CXCL10 is the key ligand for CXCR3 on CD8+ effector T cells involved in immune surveillance of the lymphocytic choriomeningitis virus-infected central nervous system. J Immunol 2006; 176(7):4235–43.

25. Rupprecht TA, Koedel U, Muhlberger B, et al. CXCL11 is involved in leucocyte recruitment to the central nervous system in neuroborreliosis. J Neurol 2005; 252(7):820–3.

26. Giunti D, Borsellino G, Benelli R, et al. Phenotypic and functional analysis of T cells homing into the CSF of subjects with inflammatory diseases of the CNS. J Leukoc Biol 2003;73(5):584–90.

27. Braitch M, Nunan R, Niepel G, et al. Increased osteopontin levels in the cerebrospinal fluid of patients with multiple sclerosis. Arch Neurol 2008;65(5):633–5.

28. Burdo TH, Ellis RJ, Fox HS. Osteopontin is increased in HIV-associated dementia. J Infect Dis 2008;198(5):715–22.

29. Chowdhury SA, Lin J, Sadiq SA. Specificity and correlation with disease activity of cerebrospinal fluid osteopontin levels in patients with multiple sclerosis. Arch Neurol 2008;65(2):232–5.

30. Mueller AM, Pedre X, Killian S, et al. The Decoy Receptor 3 (DcR3, TNFRSF6B) suppresses Th17 immune responses and is abundant in human cerebrospinal fluid. J Neuroimmunol 2009;209(1–2):57–64.

31. Yang CR, Wang JH, Hsieh SL, et al. Decoy receptor 3 (DcR3) induces osteoclast formation from monocyte/macrophage lineage precursor cells. Cell Death Differ 2004;11(Suppl 1):S97–107.

32. Hsieh CC, Lu JH, Chen SJ, et al. Cerebrospinal fluid levels of interleukin-6 and interleukin-12 in children with meningitis. Childs Nerv Syst 2009;25(4):461–5.

33. Matsuzono Y, Narita M, Akutsu Y, et al. Interleukin-6 in cerebrospinal fluid of patients with central nervous system infections. Acta Paediatr 1995;84(8):879–83.

34. Tang RB, Lee BH, Chung RL, et al. Interleukin-1beta and tumor necrosis factor-alpha in cerebrospinal fluid of children with bacterial meningitis. Childs Nerv Syst 2001;17(8):453–6.

35. Tsai ML, Chen WC, Wang YC, et al. Cerebrospinal fluid interleukin-6, interleukin-8, and tumor necrosis factor-alpha in children with central nervous system infections. Zhonghua Min Guo Xiao Er Ke Yi Xue Hui Za Zhi 1996;37(1):16–21.

36. Ichiyama T, Nishikawa M, Yoshitomi T, et al. Tumor necrosis factor-alpha, interleukin-1 beta, and interleukin-6 in cerebrospinal fluid from children with prolonged febrile seizures. Comparison with acute encephalitis/encephalopathy. Neurology 1998;50(2):407–11.

37. John CC, Panoskaltsis-Mortari A, Opoka RO, et al. Cerebrospinal fluid cytokine levels and cognitive impairment in cerebral malaria. Am J Trop Med Hyg 2008; 78(2):198–205.

38. John CC, Park GS, Sam-Agudu N, et al. Elevated serum levels of IL-1ra in children with Plasmodium falciparum malaria are associated with increased severity of disease. Cytokine 2008;41(3):204–8.

39. Lepej SZ, Misic-Majerus L, Jeren T, et al. Chemokines CXCL10 and CXCL11 in the cerebrospinal fluid of patients with tick-borne encephalitis. Acta Neurol Scand 2007;115(2):109–14.
40. Saruhan-Direskeneli G, Gurses C, Demirbilek V, et al. Elevated interleukin-12 and CXCL10 in subacute sclerosing panencephalitis. Cytokine 2005;32(2):104–10.
41. Rossi S, Studer V, Motta C, et al. Cerebrospinal fluid detection of interleukin-1beta in phase of remission predicts disease progression in multiple sclerosis. J Neuroinflammation 2014;11:32.
42. Mahad DJ, Howell SJ, Woodroofe MN. Expression of chemokines in the CSF and correlation with clinical disease activity in patients with multiple sclerosis. J Neurol Neurosurg Psychiatry 2002;72(4):498–502.
43. Bartosik-Psujek H, Stelmasiak Z. The levels of chemokines CXCL8, CCL2 and CCL5 in multiple sclerosis patients are linked to the activity of the disease. Eur J Neurol 2005;12(1):49–54.
44. Sellebjerg F, Bornsen L, Khademi M, et al. Increased cerebrospinal fluid concentrations of the chemokine CXCL13 in active MS. Neurology 2009;73(23):2003–10.
45. Mellergård J, Edstrom M, Vrethem M, et al. Natalizumab treatment in multiple sclerosis: marked decline of chemokines and cytokines in cerebrospinal fluid. Mult Scler 2010;16(2):208–17.
46. Press R, Pashenkov M, Jin JP, et al. Aberrated levels of cerebrospinal fluid chemokines in Guillain-Barre syndrome and chronic inflammatory demyelinating polyradiculoneuropathy. J Clin Immunol 2003;23(4):259–67.
47. Chen SJ, Wang YL, Kao JH, et al. Decoy receptor 3 ameliorates experimental autoimmune encephalomyelitis by directly counteracting local inflammation and downregulating Th17 cells. Mol Immunol 2009;47(2–3):567–74.
48. Kimura A, Sakurai T, Koumura A, et al. Longitudinal analysis of cytokines and chemokines in the cerebrospinal fluid of a patient with Neuro-Sweet disease presenting with recurrent encephalomeningitis. Intern Med 2008;47:135–41.
49. Hirohata S, Isshi K, Oguchi H, et al. Cerebrospinal fluid interleukin-6 in progressive Neuro-Behcet's syndrome. Clin Immunol Immunopathol 1997;82(1):12–7.
50. Townsend KP, Shytle DR, Bai Y, et al. Lovastatin modulation of microglial activation via suppression of functional CD40 expression. J Neurosci Res 2004;78(2):167–76.
51. Giunta B, Figueroa KP, Town T, et al. Soluble CD40 ligand in dementia. Drugs Future 2009;34(4):333–40.
52. McCoy MK, Tansey MG. TNF signaling inhibition in the CNS: implications for normal brain function and neurodegenerative disease. J Neuroinflammation 2008;5:45.
53. Kuhle J, Lindberg RL, Regeniter A, et al. Increased levels of inflammatory chemokines in amyotrophic lateral sclerosis. Eur J Neurol 2009;16(6):771–4.
54. Gonzalez H, Khademi M, Andersson M, et al. Prior poliomyelitis-IVIg treatment reduces proinflammatory cytokine production. J Neuroimmunol 2004;150(1–2):139–44.
55. Sharief MK, Hentges R, Ciardi M. Intrathecal immune response in patients with the post-polio syndrome. N Engl J Med 1991;325(11):749–55.
56. Colucci S, Brunetti G, Mori G, et al. Soluble decoy receptor 3 modulates the survival and formation of osteoclasts from multiple myeloma bone disease patients. Leukemia 2009;23(11):2139–46.
57. Fischer L, Korfel A, Pfeiffer S, et al. CXCL13 and CXCL12 in central nervous system lymphoma patients. Clin Cancer Res 2009;15(19):5968–73.

58. Murase S, Saio M, Andoh H, et al. Diagnostic utility of CSF soluble CD27 for primary central nervous system lymphoma in immunocompetent patients. Neurol Res 2000;22(5):434–42.
59. Fainardi E, Castellazzi M, Bellini T, et al. Cerebrospinal fluid and serum levels and intrathecal production of active matrix metalloproteinase-9 (MMP-9) as markers of disease activity in patients with multiple sclerosis. Mult Scler 2006; 12(3):294–301.
60. del Zoppo GJ, Milner R, Mabuchi T, et al. Microglial activation and matrix protease generation during focal cerebral ischemia. Stroke 2007;38(2 Suppl):646–51.
61. Pul R, Kopadze T, Skripuletz T, et al. Polyclonal immunoglobulins (IVIg) induce expression of MMP-9 in microglia. J Neuroimmunol 2009;217(1–2):46–50.
62. Mitosek-Szewczyk K, Stelmasiak Z, Bartosik-Psujek H, et al. Impact of cladribine on soluble adhesion molecules in multiple sclerosis. Acta Neurol Scand 2010;122(6):409–13.
63. Dotevall L, Hagberg L, Karlsson JE, et al. Astroglial and neuronal proteins in cerebrospinal fluid as markers of CNS involvement in Lyme neuroborreliosis. Eur J Neurol 1999;6(2):169–78.
64. Osterlundh G, Kjellmer I, Lannering B, et al. Neurochemical markers of brain damage in cerebrospinal fluid during induction treatment of acute lymphoblastic leukemia in children. Pediatr Blood Cancer 2008;50(4):793–8.
65. Kolb SA, Lahrtz F, Paul R, et al. Matrix metalloproteinases and tissue inhibitors of metalloproteinases in viral meningitis: upregulation of MMP-9 and TIMP-1 in cerebrospinal fluid. J Neuroimmunol 1998;84(2):143–50.
66. Lee KY, Kim EH, Yang WS, et al. Persistent increase of matrix metalloproteinases in cerebrospinal fluid of tuberculous meningitis. J Neurol Sci 2004;220(1–2):73–8.
67. Sulik A, Wojtkowska M, Oldak E. Elevated levels of MMP-9 and TIMP-1 in the cerebrospinal fluid of children with echovirus type 30 and mumps meningitis. Scand J Immunol 2008;68(3):323–7.
68. Matsuura E, Umehara F, Hashiguchi T, et al. Marked increase of matrix metalloproteinase 9 in cerebrospinal fluid of patients with fungal or tuberculous meningoencephalitis. J Neurol Sci 2000;173(1):45–52.
69. Hamzaoui K, Maitre B, Hamzaoui A. Elevated levels of MMP-9 and TIMP-1 in the cerebrospinal fluid of neuro-Behcet's disease. Clin Exp Rheumatol 2009;27(2 Suppl 53):S52–7.
70. Sugiyama N, Hamano S, Tanaka M, et al. A prognostic value of neuron-specific enolase in cerebrospinal fluid of acute cerebellar ataxia. Tokai J Exp Clin Med 2010;35(1):25–8.
71. Gonzalez H, Ottervald J, Nilsson KC, et al. Identification of novel candidate protein biomarkers for the post-polio syndrome - implications for diagnosis, neurodegeneration and neuroinflammation. J Proteomics 2009;71(6):670–81.
72. Rommer PS, Greilberger J, Salhofer-Polanyi S, et al. Elevated levels of carbonyl proteins in cerebrospinal fluid of patients with neurodegenerative diseases. Tohoku J Exp Med 2014;234(4):313–7.
73. Miyajima M, Nakajima M, Motoi Y, et al. Leucine-rich alpha2-glycoprotein is a novel biomarker of neurodegenerative disease in human cerebrospinal fluid and causes neurodegeneration in mouse cerebral cortex. PLoS One 2013; 8(9):e74453.
74. Gregory A, Westaway SK, Holm IE, et al. Neurodegeneration associated with genetic defects in phospholipase A(2). Neurology 2008;71(18):1402–9.
75. Matarin MM, Singleton AB, Houlden H. PANK2 gene analysis confirms genetic heterogeneity in neurodegeneration with brain iron accumulation (NBIA) but

mutations are rare in other types of adult neurodegenerative disease. Neurosci Lett 2006;407(2):162–5.

76. Grois N, Barkovich AJ, Rosenau W, et al. Central nervous system disease associated with Langerhans' cell histiocytosis. Am J Pediatr Hematol Oncol 1993; 15(2):245–54.

77. Adamus G. Autoantibody targets and their cancer relationship in the pathogenicity of paraneoplastic retinopathy. Autoimmun Rev 2009;8(5):410–4.

78. Chan KH, Vernino S, Lennon VA. ANNA-3 anti-neuronal nuclear antibody: marker of lung cancer-related autoimmunity. Ann Neurol 2001;50(3):301–11.

79. Maghnie M, Ghirardello S, De Bellis A, et al. Idiopathic central diabetes insipidus in children and young adults is commonly associated with vasopressin-cell antibodies and markers of autoimmunity. Clin Endocrinol 2006;65(4): 470–8.

80. Pivonello R, De Bellis A, Faggiano A, et al. Central diabetes insipidus and auto-immunity: relationship between the occurrence of antibodies to arginine vasopressin-secreting cells and clinical, immunological, and radiological features in a large cohort of patients with central diabetes insipidus of known and unknown etiology. J Clin Endocrinol Metab 2003;88(4):1629–36.

81. Church AJ, Dale RC, Giovannoni G. Anti-basal ganglia antibodies: a possible diagnostic utility in idiopathic movement disorders? Arch Dis Child 2004; 89(7):611–4.

82. Martino D, Giovannoni G. Antibasal ganglia antibodies and their relevance to movement disorders. Curr Opin Neurol 2004;17(4):425–32.

83. Dalmau J, Gleichman AJ, Hughes EG, et al. Anti-NMDA-receptor encephalitis: case series and analysis of the effects of antibodies. Lancet Neurol 2008; 7(12):1091–8.

84. Dalmau J, Tuzun E, Wu HY, et al. Paraneoplastic anti-N-methyl-D-aspartate receptor encephalitis associated with ovarian teratoma. Ann Neurol 2007;61(1): 25–36.

85. Malter MP, Elger CE, Surges R. Diagnostic value of CSF findings in antibody-associated limbic and anti-NMDAR-encephalitis. Seizure 2013;22(2):136–40.

86. Huda R, Tuzun E, Christadoss P. Targeting complement system to treat myasthenia gravis. Rev Neurosci 2014;25(4):575–83.

87. Kuroda H, Fujihara K, Takano R, et al. Increase of complement fragment C5a in cerebrospinal fluid during exacerbation of neuromyelitis optica. J Neuroimmunol 2013;254(1–2):178–82.

88. Wang H, Wang K, Wang C, et al. Increased soluble C5b-9 in CSF of neuromyelitis optica. Scand J Immunol 2014;79(2):127–30.

89. Pittock SJ, Lennon VA, McKeon A, et al. Eculizumab in AQP4-IgG-positive relapsing neuromyelitis optica spectrum disorders: an open-label pilot study. Lancet Neurol 2013;12(6):554–62.

90. Finehout EJ, Franck Z, Lee KH. Complement protein isoforms in CSF as possible biomarkers for neurodegenerative disease. Dis Markers 2005;21(2):93–101.

91. Toledo JB, Korff A, Shaw LM, et al. Low levels of cerebrospinal fluid complement 3 and factor H predict faster cognitive decline in mild cognitive impairment. Alzheimers Res Ther 2014;6(3):36.

92. Lleo A, Cavedo E, Parnetti L, et al. Cerebrospinal fluid biomarkers in trials for Alzheimer and Parkinson diseases. Nat Rev Neurol 2015;11(1):41–55.

93. Kang JH, Ryoo NY, Shin DW, et al. Role of cerebrospinal fluid biomarkers in clinical trials for Alzheimer's disease modifying therapies. Korean J Physiol Pharmacol 2014;18(6):447–56.

94. Jimenez-Jimenez FJ, Alonso-Navarro H, Garcia-Martin E, et al. Cerebrospinal fluid biochemical studies in patients with Parkinson's disease: toward a potential search for biomarkers for this disease. Front Cell Neurosci 2014;8:369.

95. Okonkwo OC, Alosco ML, Griffith HR, et al, Alzheimer's Disease Neuroimaging Initiative. Cerebrospinal fluid abnormalities and rate of decline in everyday function across the dementia spectrum: normal aging, mild cognitive impairment, and Alzheimer disease. Arch Neurol 2010;67(6):688–96.

96. Faull M, Ching SY, Jarmolowicz AI, et al. Comparison of two methods for the analysis of CSF Abeta and tau in the diagnosis of Alzheimer's disease. Am J Neurodegener Dis 2014;3(3):143–51.

97. O'Regan A, Berman JS. Osteopontin: a key cytokine in cell-mediated and granulomatous inflammation. Int J Exp Pathol 2000;81(6):373–90.

98. Allen CE, Li L, Peters TL, et al. Cell-specific gene expression in Langerhans cell histiocytosis lesions reveals a distinct profile compared with epidermal Langerhans cells. J Immunol 2010;184(8):4557–67.

99. Prasse A, Stahl M, Schulz G, et al. Essential role of osteopontin in smoking-related interstitial lung diseases. Am J Pathol 2009;174(5):1683–91.

100. Korn T, Bettelli E, Oukka M, et al. IL-17 and Th17 cells. Annu Rev Immunol 2009; 27:485–517.

101. Coury F, Annels N, Rivollier A, et al. Langerhans cell histiocytosis reveals a new IL-17A-dependent pathway of dendritic cell fusion. Nat Med 2008;14(1):81–7.

102. Peters TL, McClain KL, Allen CE. Neither IL-17A mRNA nor IL-17A protein are detectable in Langerhans cell histiocytosis lesions. Mol Ther 2011;19(8):1433–9.

103. Chan A, Papadimitriou C, Graf W, et al. Effects of polyclonal immunoglobulins and other immunomodulatory agents on microglial phagocytosis of apoptotic inflammatory T-cells. J Neuroimmunol 2003;135(1–2):161–5.

104. Janke AD, Yong VW. Impact of IVIg on the interaction between activated T cells and microglia. Neurol Res 2006;28(3):270–4.

105. Relkin NR, Szabo P, Adamiak B, et al. 18-Month study of intravenous immunoglobulin for treatment of mild Alzheimer disease. Neurobiol Aging 2009; 30(11):1728–36.

106. Solomon B. Intravenous immunoglobulin and Alzheimer's disease immunotherapy. Curr Opin Mol Ther 2007;9(1):79–85.

107. van Immerzeel TD, van Gilst RM, Hartwig NG. Beneficial use of immunoglobulins in the treatment of Sydenham chorea. Eur J Pediatr 2010;169(9):1151–4.

108. Gavhed D, Laurencikas E, Akefeldt SO, et al. Fifteen years of treatment with intravenous immunoglobulin in central nervous system Langerhans cell histiocytosis. Acta Paediatr 2011;100(7):e36–9.

109. Imashuku S, Fujita N, Shioda Y, et al. Follow-up of pediatric patients treated by IVIG for Langerhans cell histiocytosis (LCH)-related neurodegenerative CNS disease. Int J Hematol 2015;101(2):191–7.

110. Shioda Y, Adachi S, Imashuku S, et al. Analysis of 43 cases of Langerhans cell histiocytosis (LCH)-induced central diabetes insipidus registered in the JLSG-96 and JLSG-02 studies in Japan. Int J Hematol 2011;94(6):545–51.

111. Moravan M, Segal BM. Treatment of CNS sarcoidosis with infliximab and mycophenolate mofetil. Neurology 2009;72(4):337–40.

112. Toth C, Martin L, Morrish W, et al. Dramatic MRI improvement with refractory neurosarcoidosis treated with infliximab. Acta Neurol Scand 2007;116(4):259–62.

113. Tweedie D, Sambamurti K, Greig NH. TNF-alpha inhibition as a treatment strategy for neurodegenerative disorders: new drug candidates and targets. Curr Alzheimer Res 2007;4(4):378–85.

114. Baumann M, Cerny T, Sommacal A, et al. Langerhans cell histiocytosis with central nervous system involvement–complete response to 2-chlorodeoxyadenosine after failure of tyrosine kinase inhibitor therapies with sorafenib and imatinib. Hematol Oncol 2012;30(2):101–4.

115. Savardekar A, Tripathi M, Bansal D, et al. Isolated tumorous Langerhans cell histiocytosis of the brainstem: a diagnostic and therapeutic challenge. J Neurosurg Pediatr 2013;12(3):258–61.

116. Dhall G, Finlay JL, Dunkel IJ, et al. Analysis of outcome for patients with mass lesions of the central nervous system due to Langerhans cell histiocytosis treated with 2-chlorodeoxyadenosine. Pediatr Blood Cancer 2008;50(1):72–9.

117. Allen CE, Flores R, Rauch R, et al. Neurodegenerative central nervous system Langerhans cell histiocytosis and coincident hydrocephalus treated with vincristine/cytosine arabinoside. Pediatr Blood Cancer 2010;54(3):416–23.

118. Idbaih A, Donadieu J, Barthez MA, et al. Retinoic acid therapy in "degenerative-like" neuro-langerhans cell histiocytosis: a prospective pilot study. Pediatr Blood Cancer 2004;43(1):55–8.

119. Buchler T, Cervinek L, Belohlavek O, et al. Langerhans cell histiocytosis with central nervous system involvement: follow-up by FDG-PET during treatment with cladribine. Pediatr Blood Cancer 2005;44(3):286–8.

120. Giovannoni G, Comi G, Cook S, et al. A placebo-controlled trial of oral cladribine for relapsing multiple sclerosis. N Engl J Med 2010;362(5):416–26.

121. Hartung HP, Aktas O, Kieseier B, et al. Development of oral cladribine for the treatment of multiple sclerosis. J Neurol 2010;257(2):163–70.

122. Ottaviano F, Finlay JL. Diabetes insipidus and Langerhans cell histiocytosis: a case report of reversibility with 2-chlorodeoxyadenosine. J Pediatr Hematol Oncol 2003;25(7):575–7.

Pathogenesis of Hemophagocytic Lymphohistiocytosis

Alexandra H. Filipovich, MD,
Shanmuganathan Chandrakasan, MD*

KEYWORDS

- Pathogenesis • Hemophagocytic lymphohistiocytosis • Genetics • Secondary HLH
- Pathophysiology • Treatment

KEY POINTS

- Hemophagocytic lymphohistiocytosis (HLH), an inherited life-threatening inflammatory disorder, has gained growing recognition not only in children but also increasingly in adults over the past 2 decades.
- HLH involves inborn defects in lymphocytes (particularly in cytotoxic cells, such as natural killer [NK] cells, cytotoxic T cells, and T-regulatory cells), which normally mediate control of infectious and inflammatory conditions within the immune system and in other tissues.
- Cytotoxic cells form during hematopoietic development to include granules containing perforin and granzyme B, which are necessary to facilitate the subtle degradation of cells throughout the body, which are senescent and/or toxic to the organism.

INTRODUCTION

HLH, an inherited life-threatening inflammatory disorder, has gained growing recognition not only in children but also increasingly in adults over the past 2 decades.[1] HLH involves inborn defects in lymphocytes (particularly in cytotoxic cells, such as NK cells, cytotoxic T cells, and T-regulatory cells), which normally mediate control of infectious and inflammatory conditions within the immune system and in other tissues.[2]

Cytotoxic cells form during hematopoietic development to include granules containing perforin and granzyme B, which are necessary to facilitate the subtle degradation of cells throughout the body, which are senescent and/or toxic to the organism.[3]

In the context of inherited defects in cytotoxic cells and other immune cells, the disorder is classified as familial HLH (FHLH) or primary HLH. Secondary HLH occurs in

Immunodeficiency and Histiocytosis Program, Cancer and Blood Diseases Institute, Cincinnati Children's Hospital Medical Center, 3333 Burnet Avenue, Cincinnati, OH 45229-3039, USA
* Corresponding author.
E-mail address: Shanmuganathan.Chandrakasan@cchmc.org

Hematol Oncol Clin N Am 29 (2015) 895–902
http://dx.doi.org/10.1016/j.hoc.2015.06.007
0889-8588/15/$ – see front matter © 2015 Elsevier Inc. All rights reserved.

the settings of infections (eg, Epstein-Barr virus [EBV] infections) or underlying rheumatologic disorders (often described as macrophage activation syndrome [MAS]). Secondary HLH also accompanies some lymphoid malignancies.

DISEASE DESCRIPTION

In patients with FHLH, inborn defects of lymphocyte cytotoxicity lead to ineffective infection control and immune dysregulation.[4] Patients with FHLH are likely to manifest the clinical disorder in childhood, on rare occasion with symptoms noted in utero. This immune activation is manifested by abnormally high levels of predominantly proinflammatory cytokines, including interferon gamma and interleukins (ILs) IL-1, IL-6, and the compensatory down-regulating cytokine IL-10.

Consequent clinical findings include high-grade fevers, progressive cytopenias, coagulopathy, and a broad spectrum of neurologic symptoms, including seizures and altered sensorium. More recently, there has been a wider recognition that fulminant liver failure may be an early and rapidly evolving presentation of HLH; swift immunosuppressive and anti-inflammatory treatment can occasionally obviate emergency liver allograft.

The first documented description of what is now called HLH was published by Farquhar and Claireux[5] at the University of Edinburgh in 1952. They recognized the constellation of signs and symptoms noted in a brother and sister healthy at birth, who developed recurrent unexplained fevers, "progressive panhematopenia," hepatosplenomegaly, and bruising noted in the 3rd month of life. At autopsy, both children manifested "inflammatory cell infiltration"; mainly lymphocytes and plasma cells were found, many of which manifested erythrophagocytosis and cells in the liver and "highly reactive marrow." A "great proliferation of histiocytes" was found; "many of these histiocytes showed erythrophagocytosis and others contained lymphocytes and polymorphs."

Diagnostic criteria for HLH have been developed and reviewed more recently by the Histiocyte Society[6] (**Box 1**). The most prevalent early findings include fevers (persistent or frequent), cytopenias typically involving 2 or more lineages, and liver dysfunction. Hemophagocytosis in the bone marrow, cerebrospinal fluid, or other sites in the context of aforementioned symptoms suggest a strong probability of active HLH. The likelihood is greatly strengthened by the coincident detection of high levels of the inflammatory molecules: ferritin and soluble IL-2 receptor (age dependent) in the blood. Splenomegaly may be palpable or may be observed radiologically. These features are seen in children and adults.[7]

One of the more problematic diagnostic criteria recommended by the Histiocyte Society is quantitation of NK cell function. Classic NK cytotoxic assays assume that the proportion of circulating NK cells is in normal range in the blood sample; this is not always known. More quantitative studies include quantitation of the perforin expression within NK cells and the degranulation assay (testing active function of NK cells); these assays should only be sent to certified laboratories that perform significant numbers of such assays.

GENETICS OF HEMOPHAGOCYTIC LMPHOHISTIOCYTOSIS

To date, 12 distinct genetic disorders resulting in HLH have been defined; 9 disorders are expressed due to biallelic autosomal recessive gene defects, whereas 3 are X-linked. Importantly, 10 of the genetic defects can be rapidly screened for by flow cytometry assays (**Fig. 1, Table 1**).

Box 1
Diagnostic criteria for hemophagocytic lymphohistiocytosis (≥5 of the 8 criteria)

1. Fever

2. Splenomegaly

3. Cytopenias (affecting 2 of 3 lineages in the peripheral blood)

   a. Hemoglobin less than 90 g/L (in infants <4 weeks: hemoglobin <100 g/L)

   b. Platelets less than 100 × 10⁹/L

   c. Neutrophils less than 1.0 × 10⁹/L

4. Hypertriglyceridemia and/or hypofibrinogenemia

   a. Fasting triglycerides greater than 3.0 mmol/L

   b. Fibrinogen less than 1.5 g/L

5. Hemophagocytosis in bone marrow or spleen or lymph nodes

6. Low or absent NK-cell activity

7. Ferritin greater than 500 μg/L

8. Soluble IL-2 receptor greater than 2400 U/mL

Adapted from Henter JI, Horne A, Aricó M, et al. HLH-2004: diagnostic and therapeutic guidelines for hemophagocytic lymphohistiocytosis. Pediatr Blood Cancer 2007;48(2):126; with permission.

The first genetic defect defined in association with HLH was perforin deficiency. Perforin is a cytolytic mediator produced by killer lymphocytes packaged and ultimately released from cytoplasmic granules when the effector cells are activated. Perforin is partially homologous to the terminal components of the membrane attack complex, producing porelike lesions up to 20 nm in diameter on target cell membranes on activation. The effector molecule, granzyme B, a serine protease also found in cytolytic cells, is delivered into target cells (predominantly cancerous or pathogen infected cells) via the porelike structures, which are generated on activation of NK cells and cytotoxic T cells. Broadly, granzyme B then induces programmed cell death in target cells (**Fig. 2**).

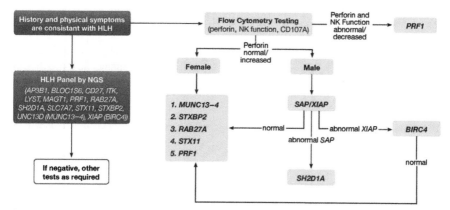

Fig. 1. FHL diagnostic algorithm. If absolute lymphocyte count less than 300 cells/μL, proceed to sequencing in lieu of flow cytometry testing. Saliva is preferred method of sample collection in patients with white blood cell counts less than 2000 cells/μL.

Table 1
Classification of primary hemophagocytic lymphohistiocytosis, notable clinical findings, and rapid diagnostic methods

Hemophagocytic Lymphohistiocytosis Type	Gene	Function	Notable Clinical Findings	Rapid Diagnosis by Flow Cytometry
FHLH-1	Unknown	NA	—	NA
FHLH-2	PRF1	Pore formation	—	Decreased/absent perforin expression
FHLH-3	UNC13D	Vesicle priming	Increased incidence of central nervous system HLH	Decreased CD107a expression
FHLH-4	STX11	Vesicle fusion	Mild and recurrent HLH and colitis	Decreased CD107a expression
FHLH-5	STXBP2	Vesicle fusion	Colitis, bleeding tendency, and hypogammaglobulinemia	Decreased CD107a expression
Syndromes				
Griscelli syndrome type II	RAB27A	Vesicle docking	Partial albinism and silvery-gray hair	Decreased CD 107a expression, abnormal hair shaft examination[a]
Chédiak–Higashi syndrome	LYST	Vesicle trafficking	Partial albinism, bleeding tendency, and recurrent pyogenic infection	Decreased CD 107a expression, abnormal neutrophil granules[b]
Hermansky-Pudlak syndrome type II	AP3B1	Vesicle trafficking	Partial albinism, bleeding tendency, and immunodeficiency	Decreased CD 107a expression
EBV driven				
XLP-1	SH2D1A	Signaling in T, NK, and NK T cells	Hypogammaglobulinemia and lymphoma	Decreased/absent SAP expression
XLP-2/XIAP[c]	BIRC4	Signaling pathways involving nuclear factor κB	Mild and recurrent HLH and colitis	Decreased/absent XIAP expression
ITK deficiency	ITK	Signaling in T-cell pathways	AR and Hodgkin lymphoma	NA (gene sequencing)
CD27 deficiency	CD27	Lymphocyte costimulatory molecule	AR and combined immunodeficiency	Absent CD27 expression on B cells
XMEN	MAGT1	T-cell activation via T-cell receptor	Combined immunodeficiency, severe chronic viral infections, and lymphoma	Decreased CD4 cells and defects in T-cell receptor signaling

Abbreviations: AR, autosomal recessive; *MAGT1*, magnesium transporter 1; NA, not available; XIAP, X-linked inhibitor of apoptosis protein; XLP, X-linked lymphoproliferative; XMEN, X-linked immunodeficiency with Mg(2+) defect, EBV infection, and neoplasia.
[a] Light microscopy examination of a hair shaft shows a characteristic abnormal clumping of pigment.
[b] Light microscopy examination of peripheral blood smear shows giant granules in neutrophils and other leukocytes.
[c] Defect is present in all tissues.

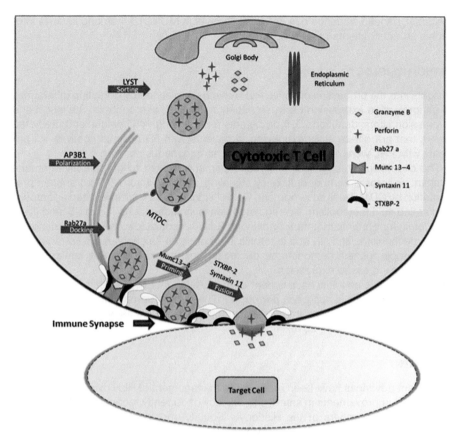

Fig. 2. Degranulation pathway in cytotoxic T lymphocyte and function of different proteins associated with known HLH defects. (*Adapted from* Chandrakasan S, Filipovich AH. Hemophagocytic lymphohistiocytosis: advances in pathophysiology, diagnosis, and treatment. J Pediatr 2013;163(5):1254)

Five other HLH-related syndromes are associated with vesicle priming, fusion, docking, or trafficking (see **Table 1**). Three diseases that can lead to HLH-like reactions are X-linked (see **Table 1**) and all 3 have a propensity to development of HLH-like symptoms after exposure to EBV. Other symptoms frequently seen in the X-linked disorders include immunodeficiency (most often hypogammaglobulinemia or dysgammaglobulinemia.), colitis, and lymphoproliferative disorders.[8] Much rarer recently described disorders related to persistent or recurrent EBV infection include IL-2–inducible T-cell kinase (ITK) deficiency and CD27 deficiency.

SECONDARY HEMOPHAGOCYTIC LYMPHOHISTIOCYTOSIS

Infections and rheumatologic conditions are the 2 most common contributors to secondary HLH in children and adults. Infectious mononucleosis can mimic most features of HLH, and EBV infection is the most common trigger. Additionally, in endemic areas HLH may be confused with leishmaniasis.

MAS, or the accelerated phase of rheumatologic disorders, especially juvenile rheumatoid arthritis and lupus erythematosus, mimics many of the features of classic HLH.

Recently, genetic evidence has detected variants in MUNC13-4 among juvenile idiopathic arthritis patients presenting with MAS.[9,10]

PATHOPHYSIOLOGY

Insights into the processes of active HLH have been gleaned by detecting differences in genome-wide expression between patients with FHL and controls. Statistical and expression filters identified 2054 probe sets representing 1465 unique and predicted genes that are differentially expressed in patients with FHL versus controls. All patients with FHL were clustered together in a homogeneous manner.[11]

The down-regulated genes were found primarily related to the adaptive immune system, apoptosis, immunodeficiency signaling, nuclear factor κB, lipid antigen presentation by CD1, B-cell development, CTLA4 signaling, calcium-mediated apoptosis, and amino acid metabolism. Up-regulated genes included IL-10, IL-6, IL-8, and IL-17 (predominantly proinflammatory cytokines). Genes associated with innate immune defense mechanisms and NK and cytotoxic T lymphocyte function are down-regulated. Proapoptopic genes demonstrate decreased expression whereas antiapoptotic genes have increased expression.

More recently, an initial assessment of microRNAs (miRNAs) in samples from patients with active HLH has been performed. The 6 most up-regulated miRNAs were found associated with other immune/inflammatory disorders as well (Janos Sumegi, personal communication, 2015).

TREATMENT

Significant advances have been made in the management of HLH over the past 2 decades.[12,13] Improvements in safety and efficacy of currently recommended therapies have involved members of the Histiocyte Society and other HLH-focused groups around the world, including corporate investigators. Current management of HLH recommended by the Histiocyte Society involves a 2-step approach. The first phase involves gaining control of the inflammatory process, ideally by destroying the infectious trigger if present, followed by reducing T-cell activation and proliferation through the use of steroids, etoposide and anti–T-cell agents. International protocols developed by the Histiocyte Society have reported a remission induction rate of 71%, and 5-year post-transplant survival probability of 54% ± 6%. Patients whose HLH was well controlled at the time of allogeneic stem cell transplantation experienced better long-term outcomes. More recently, an HLH protocol (reduced intensity chemotherapy [RIC]) using alemtuzumab (a monoclonal antibody targeting CD52 on mature lymphocytes while sparing the stem cells), delivered 2 weeks prior to the infusion of donor cells,[14,15] has improved outcomes. This clinical protocol has yielded the best transplant outcomes for HLH to date (**Fig. 3**).

French investigators have tested a protocol combining front-line antithymocyte globulin (ATG) in combination with steroids, yielding an 82% short-term clinical response. Based on the apparent efficacy of ATG, a protocol including ATG, named hybrid immunotherapy for HLH, has been opened in the United States.

The most promising novel induction therapy, which can be used as frontline therapy or on HLH reactivation, is a humanized antibody that targets gamma interferon. The concept was first tested in a murine model of HLH. It has been learned that gamma interferon is found elevated in most patients at onset of HLH as well as reactivation of HLH. The first treatment study developed by a Swiss company, Novimmune, shows promise in an early human trial.

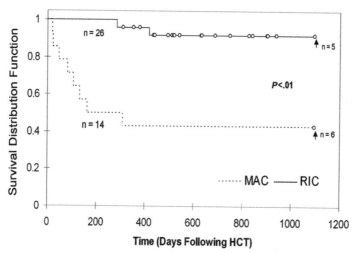

Fig. 3. Kaplan-Meier 3-year survival curves for the MAC and RIC groups. (*From* Marsh RA, Vaughn G, Kim MO, et al. Reduced-intensity conditioning significantly improves survival of patients with hemophagocytic lymphohistiocytosis undergoing allogeneic hematopoietic cell transplantation. Blood 2010;116:5830; with permission; © 2010 by American Society of Hematology.)

REFERENCES

1. Janka GE. Familial hemophagocytic lymphohistiocytosis. Eur J Pediatr 1983; 140(3):221–30.
2. Ladisch S, Poplack DG, Holiman B, et al. Immunodeficiency in familial erythro-phagocytic lymphohistiocytosis. Lancet 1978;1(8064):581–3.
3. Lykens JE, Terrell CE, Zoller EE, et al. Perforin is a critical physiologic regulator of T-cell activation. Blood 2011;118(3):618–26.
4. Henter JI, Elinder G, Söder O, et al. Hypercytokinemia in familial hemophagocytic lymphohistiocytosis. Blood 1991;78(11):2918–22.
5. Farquhar JW, Claireaux AE. Familial haemophagocytic reticulosis. Arch Dis Child 1952;27(136):519–25.
6. Henter JI, Horne A, Aricó M, et al. HLH-2004: diagnostic and therapeutic guidelines for hemophagocytic lymphohistiocytosis. Pediatr Blood Cancer 2007;48(2):124–31.
7. Raschke RA, Garcia-Orr R. Hemophagocytic lymphohistiocytosis: a potentially underrecognized association with systemic inflammatory response syndrome, severe sepsis, and septic shock in adults. Chest 2011;140(4):933–8.
8. Pachlopnik Schmid J, Canioni D, Moshous D, et al. Clinical similarities and differences of patients with X-linked lymphoproliferative syndrome type 1 (XLP-1/SAP deficiency) versus type 2 (XLP-2/XIAP deficiency). Blood 2011;117(5):1522–9.
9. Zhang K, Biroschak J, Glass DN, et al. Macrophage activation syndrome in patients with systemic juvenile idiopathic arthritis is associated with MUNC13-4 polymorphisms. Arthritis Rheum 2008;58(9):2892–6.
10. Sumegi J, Barnes MG, Nestheide SV, et al. Gene expression profiling of peripheral blood mononuclear cells from children with active hemophagocytic lymphohistiocytosis. Blood 2011;117(15):e151–60.
11. Henter JI, Samuelsson-Horne A, Aricò M, et al. Treatment of hemophagocytic lymphohistiocytosis with HLH-94 immunochemotherapy and bone marrow transplantation. Blood 2002;100(7):2367–73.

12. Jordan MB, Allen CE, Weitzman S, et al. How I treat hemophagocytic lymphohistiocytosis. Blood 2011;118(15):4041–52.

13. Zhang K, Jordan MB, Marsh RA, et al. Hypomorphic mutations in PRF1, MUNC13-4, and STXBP2 are associated with adult-onset familial HLH. Blood 2011;118(22):5794–8.

14. Marsh RA, Vaughn G, Kim MO, et al. Reduced-intensity conditioning significantly improves survival of patients with hemophagocytic lymphohistiocytosis undergoing allogeneic hematopoietic cell transplantation. Blood 2010;116(26):5824–31.

15. Cooper N, Rao K, Gilmour K, et al. Stem cell transplantation with reduced-intensity conditioning for hemophagocytic lymphohistiocytosis. Blood 2006; 107(3):1233–6.

Familial Hemophagocytic Lymphohistiocytosis

Barbara Degar, MD[a,b]

KEYWORDS

- Hemophagocytic lymphohistiocytosis
- Familial hemophagocytic lymphohistiocytosis • HLH • FHL • Perforin • XLP

KEY POINTS

- Familial hemophagocytic lymphohistiocytosis (FHL) is a rare hyperinflammatory condition that is genetically heterogeneous. FHL is typically diagnosed in infancy but may present much later in life.
- Approximately 70% of individuals diagnosed with FHL have mutations identified in a hemophagocytic lymphohistiocytosis (HLH)–associated gene.
- FHL bears resemblance to secondary forms of HLH, including Epstein-Barr virus–associated HLH and macrophage activation syndrome. The approach to initial treatment is similar.
- Hematopoietic cell transplantation is necessary to cure FHL. Reduced-intensity conditioning before transplantation is associated with lower risk of toxicity and higher likelihood of survival.

INTRODUCTION

Familial hemophagocytic lymphohistiocytosis (FHL) is a rare, life-threatening, inherited hyperinflammatory syndrome that may be clinically indistinguishable from secondary forms of hemophagocytic lymphohistiocytosis (HLH). The molecular basis of FHL is heterogeneous, with defects occurring in 1 or more of several proteins that participate in lymphocyte cytotoxicity. In most but not all cases of FHL, the genetic defect responsible for the disease can be identified. However, in some cases, the diagnosis of FHL is presumed from a relapsing or unremitting course or a positive family history. There is still much more to be learned about the interplay between genetics and environmental factors that underlie FHL.

[a] Harvard Medical School, Harvard University, 25 Shattuck st., Boston, MA 02115, USA;
[b] Pediatric Oncology, Dana-Farber/Boston Children's Cancer and Blood Disorders Center, 450 Brookline Avenue, Boston, MA 02215, USA
E-mail address: barbara_degar@dfci.harvard.edu

Hematol Oncol Clin N Am 29 (2015) 903–913
http://dx.doi.org/10.1016/j.hoc.2015.06.008
0889-8588/15/$ – see front matter © 2015 Elsevier Inc. All rights reserved.

hemonc.theclinics.com

INCIDENCE

FHL is estimated to affect approximately 1 in 50,000 live births or 0.12 to 0.15 per 100,000 children per year.[1] The disease occurs worldwide among all races and ethnic groups. The absolute frequency of disease-causing mutations in specific HLH-associated genes varies among populations. A slight male preponderance may be attributable to the occurrence of FHL in association with X-linked lymphoproliferative disorders (XLPs).

FHL is a conditional disease in the sense that affected individuals are healthy until they encounter a trigger, such as an ordinary viral infection. Once initiated, the cycle of inflammation and the signs and symptoms that are elicited usually progress very rapidly. Secondary HLH is more prevalent than FHL; however, the true incidence of secondary HLH in children and adults remains undefined.[2]

FAMILIAL HEMOPHAGOCYTIC LYMPHOHISTIOCYTOSIS SUBTYPES

FHL was first described in 1952 in 2 infant brothers[3] and was recognized as a rare, fatal familial disease with an autosomal recessive inheritance pattern. It was not until 1999 that Stepp and colleagues[4] discovered the association of FHL with mutations in the perforin gene, establishing the molecular basis for FHL-2. In the years since, the molecular basis for FHL-3, FLH-4, and FHL-5 has been determined. The gene responsible for FHL-1, which is linked to chromosome 9q22,[5] remains a mystery. In addition, 2 distinct X-linked syndromes, XLP-1 and XLP-2, are typically associated with HLH and individuals with Griscelli syndrome, Chédiak-Higashi syndrome, Hermansky-Pudlak syndrome, and certain glycogen storage disorders sometimes develop HLH.

The underlying defect in patients with FHL can be ascribed to a defect in the primary cytotoxicity effector pathway in lymphocytes and natural killer (NK) cells, leading to poor clearance of target cells and a perpetual state of immune activation (**Fig. 1**). The genetic variants of FHL are presented in **Table 1**.

Perforin is a critical component of cytotoxic granules in effector T and NK cells. Upon effector cell degranulation, perforin and granzymes are released from the cytotoxic granules in close proximity to a target cell, such as a virally infected cell. Perforin creates a pore in the membrane of the target cell, allowing granzymes to initiate target cell death by apoptosis. Abnormal or absent perforin function leads to impaired killing of target cells and uncontrolled T-cell activation and high levels of inflammatory cytokines. This so-called cytokine storm is responsible for the tissue damage and clinical symptoms seen in HLH. Interferon (IFN) gamma is an essential player in this cascade. Blockade of IFN gamma activity using a neutralizing antibody abrogates the clinical features of HLH in perforin-deficient mice.[6]

The median age of onset of FHL-2 is 3 months. However, there is a wide range of disease onset and severity that correlates with the degree of perforin deficiency. Residual cytotoxic function and later age of onset are observed in patients with at least 1 missense mutation.[7] Among African Americans, FHL-2 accounts for most FHL cases. The 50delT is the most common mutation observed in this population and is associated with profound perforin deficiency and early disease onset.[8]

The process of effector cell cytotoxicity depends on the regulated transport, docking, priming, and fusion of perforin-containing lytic granules at the effector–target cell interface. Munc13-4 participates in preparing lytic vesicles that are docked at the cell surface for fusion with the membrane. Impaired lymphocyte cytotoxicity results from Munc13-4 deficiency[9] and biallelic mutation in Munc13-4 causes FHL-3. Disease-causing Munc13-4 mutations, which may be classified as nonsense, missense, or

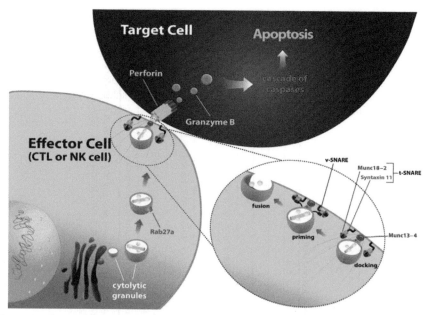

Fig. 1. Mechanics of cytotoxic function revealed by HLH-associated gene mutations. CTL, Cytotoxic T Lymphocyte. (*From* Jordan MB, Allen CE, Weitzman S, et al. How I treat hemophagocytic lymphohistiocytosis. Blood 2011;118:4044; with permission.)

both, are scattered throughout the gene. Earlier age at onset is associated with biallelic missense mutation and a more severe impairment of Munc13-4 function.[10] FHL-3 occurs in patients of all ethnicities. Although the median age of onset is 4 months, there is wide variability. Central nervous system (CNS) manifestations are especially frequent in this FHL subtype.[11]

Mutations in the putative vesicular SNAP, syntaxin-11 (STX11), are responsible for FHL-4.[12] STX11 associates with syntaxin-binding protein 2 (STXBP2/Munc18-2), regulating the fusion of lytic granules with the plasma membrane at the interface between effector and target cells. FHL-4 was first identified among Turkish/Kurdish families and is rare outside that population.

The binding of STX11 with STXBP2 regulates granule docking and initiation of SNARE complex formation. Mutations in STXBP2, also known as Munc18-2, are responsible for FHL-5.[13] The age of onset of FHL-5 is highly variable and the disease is often associated with colitis, hearing loss, and abnormal bleeding.[14]

X-linked lymphoproliferative disorders 1 and 2 are distinct X-linked syndromes characterized by susceptibility to Epstein-Barr virus (EBV) infection, HLH, and dysgammaglobulinemia. Patients with XLP-1 harbor hemizygous mutations in the Src homology 2 domain–containing gene 1A (*SH2D1A*), which functions as a lymphocyte signaling adapter.[15] These patients have a multifactorial humoral and cellular immune deficiency that, in addition to HLH and dysgammaglobulinemia, is associated with an increased risk of lymphoid malignancy. XLP-2 has been described more recently and results from mutations in the *BIRC4* gene, which encodes X-linked inhibitor of apoptosis (XIAP).[16,17] Patients with XIAP deficiency may present with colitis in addition to susceptibility to EBV infection and HLH, but they do not seem to be at increased risk for malignancy.[18]

Table 1
The genetic variants of FHL

Disease	Locus	Gene/Gene Symbol	Function	Syndromic Associations	Relative Frequency (%)
FHL-1	9q22.1-23	Unknown	—	None	—
FHL-2	10q22	Perforin/PRF1	Induction of apoptosis	None	20–30
FHL-3	17q25	Munc13-4/UNC13D	Vesicle priming	None	20–30
FHL-4	6q24	Syntaxin-11/STX11	Vesicle transport	None	<5
FHL-5	19p13	Munc18-2/STXBP2	Vesicle trafficking and release	Colitis, bleeding tendency, hearing loss	20
GS2	15q21	RAS-associated protein/RAB27A	Signal transduction	Partial albinism	—
CHS	1q42.1-42.2	Lysosomal trafficking regulator/LYST	Vesicle transport	Partial albinism, susceptibility to infection, neuropathy	—
XLP-1	Xq25	SAP/SHD2D1A	Signal transduction	Sensitivity to EBV infection, hypogammaglobulinemia, lymphoma	—
XLP-2	Xq25	XIAP/BIRC4	Induction of apoptosis	Splenomegaly, hypogammaglobulinemia	—

Abbreviations: CHS, Chédiak-Higashi syndrome; EBV, Epstein-Barr virus; GS2, Griscelli Type 2; SAP, SLAM-associated protein; XIAP, X-linked inhibitor of apoptosis.
Data from Hemophagocytic Lymphohistiocytosis, Familial, KeJian Zhang, MD, MBA, Alexandra H Filipovich, MD, Judith Johnson, MS, Rebecca A Marsh, MD, and Joyce Villanueva, MT, MBA. Gene Reviews: Initial Posting: March 22, 2006; Last Update: January 17, 2013.

Griscelli syndrome type 2 (GS2) and Chédiak-Higashi syndrome type 1 (CHS1) are autosomal recessive gene defects characterized by partial albinism in association with HLH. The GS2 protein, RAB27A, a small GTPase of the RAS-associated family, directly associates with the FHL-3 protein, Munc13-4, and participates in cytotoxic granule exocytosis.[19] HLH occurs in patients with GS2 but not in patients with GS1 or GS3, which are caused by mutations in myosin-Va and melanophilin, respectively. In melanocytes, Rab27a, melanophilin, and myosin-Va are all required for distribution of pigment-containing melanosomes. However, melanophilin and myosin-Va are not required for lymphocyte cytotoxicity. Pigmentary defects may be subtle or inapparent in patients with GS2, especially those with fair skin.[20] Like GS2, CHS is characterized by pigmentation defects, and is caused by mutations in the LYST protein, which is involved in lysosomal transport and vesicular trafficking.

Historically, FHL has been understood to be an autosomal recessive disease with high penetrance that presents in early infancy and is inevitably fatal without hematopoietic cell transplantation (HCT). However, recent and ongoing work on the molecular genetics and pathophysiology of HLH provides evidence that FHL is more varied than was once assumed. Genetic lesions in 1 or more HLH-associated genes are present in a high proportion of cases of adolescent-onset and adult-onset HLH; sequence variants in PRF1, Munc13-4, and STXBP2 were found in 25 (14%) of 175 adults with HLH who were studied retrospectively.[21] Certain monoallelic mutations, such as one illustrative case affecting STXPB2,[22] may be sufficient to impair lymphocyte cytotoxicity and contribute to HLH. In addition, synergistic defects in 2 (or more) distinct molecules involved in the cytotoxic pathway also can lead to HLH in some cases.[23] Impaired cytotoxicity related to a genetic lesion in an HLH-associated gene seems to predispose to the development of macrophage activation syndrome in some patients with rheumatologic conditions.[24]

DIAGNOSTIC WORK-UP

Diagnostic criteria for HLH were developed[25] and later updated[26] by the Histiocyte Society. Patients must fulfill at least 5 of 8 clinical and laboratory criteria, including fever, cytopenias, splenomegaly, hypertriglyceridemia and/or hypofibrinogenemia, hyperferritinemia, increased soluble CD25 (sCD25) level, depressed or absent NK cell function, and evidence of hemophagocytosis in tissue biopsy (**Box 1**). Several additional clinical and laboratory characteristics support the diagnosis, including hyponatremia, liver dysfunction, CNS symptoms, and/or abnormal cerebrospinal fluid. A documented genetic mutation, a positive family history of HLH, and parental consanguinity also strongly support the diagnosis of FHL in the presence of any of the clinical or laboratory features.

Distinguishing FHL from secondary HLH is often challenging. Documentation of biallelic pathologic mutations in an HLH-associated gene is the gold-standard diagnostic test. Sequencing of a panel of HLH-associated genes should be sent off as soon as the diagnosis is suspected. However, these studies take weeks to complete. In addition, although most cases of FHL can be molecularly verified, some familial cases still elude molecular diagnosis. In addition, interpretation of gene studies is not always straightforward because, as described earlier, apparent monoallelic mutations and synergistic mutations in distinct genes and may cause FHL.

Some specialized tests, which are not universally available, may rapidly aid in diagnosis of FHL. These studies complement gene sequencing studies.

> **Box 1**
> **Diagnostic guidelines (2004)**
>
> Molecular diagnosis consistent with HLH
>
>   Or 5 of the following 8 clinical, laboratory, and histopathologic criteria
>
> Clinical criteria
>
> - Fever
> - Splenomegaly
>
> Laboratory criteria
>
> - Cytopenias (hemoglobin level <9 g/L; platelet level <100 × 109/L; neutrophil level <1.0 × 109/L)
> - Hypertriglyceridemia and/or hypofibrinogenemia (fasting triglyceride level ≥3 standard deviations [SD], fibrinogen level ≤3 SD of normal for age)
> - Hyperferritinemia (>500 μg/L)
> - Increased CD25 level (≥2400 U/L)
> - Low/absent NK function
>
> Histopathologic criteria
>
> - Hemophagocytosis in marrow, spleen, or lymph nodes with no evidence of malignancy
>
> *From* Henter JI, Horne A, Arico M, et al. HLH-2004: diagnostic and therapeutic guidelines for hemophagocytic lymphohistiocytosis. Pediatr Blood Cancer 2007;48:126; with permission.

Flow Cytometry

Using multiparameter flow cytometry, surface expression of perforin/granzyme B and SLAM-associated protein (SAP) and intracellular expression of XIAP are measured. Determination of SAP and XIAP levels is especially valuable in the rapid identification of male patients with XLP-1 and XLP-2, respectively.

Natural Killer Function

NK cells obtained from peripheral blood mononuclear cells are assayed for the ability to lyse chromium-loaded target cells. In the setting of active HLH, the functional activity of NK cells is usually impaired.[27] An inability to reconstitute NK functional activity in vitro using modified assay conditions, and the persistence of depressed NK cell function after treatment of HLH, are associated with FHL.[28]

CD107a

When stimulated, cytotoxic T cells and NK cells undergo exocytosis, and CD107a expression is induced on the cell surface, where it can be detected by flow cytometry. If the NK cells are incapable of degranulation because of an intrinsic defect in the cytotoxic pathway, CD107a expression is diminished or absent. Importantly, this assay is normal in patients with perforin deficiency (FHL-2), XLP, and secondary HLH.[29] The CD107a degranulation assay, combined with flow cytometry for perforin, and SAP and XIAP in male patients, allows rapid identification of some patients with FHL.[30]

TREATMENT

Treatment of FHL is divided into 2 phases: (1) immune suppression to achieve and maintain control of the hyperinflammatory state, and (2) allogeneic HCT to replace the defective immune system. Those patients who are proved to harbor a disease-causing mutation in an HLH-associated gene, who fail to respond completely to initial therapy, or who experience reactivation of disease after transient resolution are presumed to have FHL and are referred for HCT. The remaining cases of presumed secondary HLH may discontinue immune suppression.

INITIAL THERAPY FOR FAMILIAL HEMOPHAGOCYTIC LYMPHOHISTIOCYTOSIS

Initial management of FHL is intended to interrupt the cycle of hyperinflammation. Typically, whether a patient has FHL or secondary HLH at initial presentation. Often, treatment is urgently needed, even if diagnostic criteria are not yet fulfilled. Without therapy, FHL is rapidly and invariably fatal, usually within a month or two of presentation.[31] The importance of supportive care, including the identification of potentially treatable infections, should never be underestimated.

In 1980, Ambruso and colleagues[32] first reported the successful treatment of 2 infants with presumed FHL with etoposide (VP-16), a cancer chemotherapy drug that is now widely used. Etoposide shows especially potent cytotoxicity against activated T cells, which may account for its efficacy in HLH.[33] The combination of etoposide and dexamethasone has been established as the standard of care for the treatment of HLH based on the results of HLH-94, a prospective, international clinical trial conducted by the Histiocyte Society. The treatment schedule is shown in **Fig. 2**. The HLH-94 study enrolled 249 eligible children between 1994 and 2003. Overall, 86% of HLH-94 participants responded to 8 weeks of initial therapy, approximately 60% of whom achieved nonactive disease.[34] To build on these favorable results, the Histiocyte Society initiated a successor study, HLH-2004 protocol, in which cyclosporine (CSA) was added during the first 8 weeks of initial therapy.[26] Preliminary results suggest that adding CSA first does not dramatically accelerate or improve the rate of response observed in HLH-94.

Alternative treatments using antibody-based approaches are designed to directly inhibit activated T cells or the inflammatory cytokines they secrete. The combination of antithymocyte globulin (ATG), dexamethasone, and CSA is a strategy championed by clinical investigators in France. Among 38 children with confirmed FHL who received 1 or 2 courses of rabbit ATG, complete resolution was achieved in 73% and partial improvement in 24%.[35] Alemtuzumab is a therapeutic monoclonal antibody that is directed against CD52, an antigen expressed on lymphocytes, NK cells, monocytes,

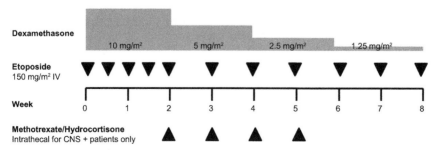

Fig. 2. Initial therapy for HLH. Based on the HLH-94 study. CNS+, CNS positive, IV, intravenous. (*Adapted from* Jordan MB, Allen CE, Weitzman S, et al. How I treat hemophagocytic lymphohistiocytosis. Blood 2011;118:4047; with permission.)

and macrophages. Alemtuzumab has not yet been studied in the initial treatment of HLH but it is effective as a bridge to transplant in patients with refractory FHL.[36] Neutralization of IFN gamma activity using a monoclonal antibody is another approach in development, but experience with this is thus far extremely limited.

CNS manifestations, including neurologic symptoms, abnormal CSF, or both, are reported in up to 63% of children with FHL at diagnosis.[37] Prompt and aggressive initiation of immunosuppression followed by HCT is the best strategy for minimizing the potential for CNS damage in FHL.[1,38] The role of CNS-directed therapy is not well established. In HLH-94, intrathecal methotrexate was administered to patients in whom neurologic symptoms progressed or CSF abnormalities did not resolve after 2 weeks of systemic treatment.

Ideally, patients with FHL should undergo HCT as soon as inflammation is controlled and a suitable stem cell donor is identified. Control of the clinical signs of HLH before transplantation significantly improves the likelihood of a successful outcome.[39]

HEMATOPOIETIC CELL TRANSPLANTATION

The first successful matched sibling donor bone marrow transplant in a boy with FHL was described in 1986.[40] Hematopoietic cell transplantation (HCT) is now routinely performed and it remains the only curative therapy for patients with FHL. Among the patients treated on the HLH-94 trial, overall survival at 5 years among the 124 patient who underwent HCT was 66%. No patients with verified FHL survived without HCT.[34]

Allogeneic transplant in patients with FHL using conventional myeloablative conditioning is associated with an excessively high rate of toxicity and death.[41] Roughly one-third of recipients of transplants after myeloablative conditioning die within the first few months after transplantation of infection, hepatopathy, pneumonitis, and/or uncontrolled disease.[6] Reduced-intensity conditioning with alemtuzumab, fludarabine, and melphalan has shown superior outcomes.[42,43] However, mixed-donor chimerism is a common obstacle and donor lymphocyte infusion is indicated in many cases. For this reason, reduced-intensity conditioning is not ideal for patients in whom the only acceptable donor source is umbilical cord blood.

SUMMARY/FUTURE DIRECTIONS

FHL is a genetically and clinically heterogeneous disorder characterized by impaired cellular cytotoxicity and uncontrolled inflammation. The clinical and laboratory features of the disorder are the result of the hyperinflammatory state. The current standard treatment of FHL is the combination of etoposide and dexamethasone, with intrathecal chemotherapy in selected cases. Currently under development are noncytotoxic inhibitors of the inflammatory response that have the potential to effectively treat HLH without causing myelosuppression or an increased risk of malignancy. Presently, FHL can only be cured by HCT. HCT using reduced-intensity conditioning is associated with a superior outcome compared with myeloablative conditioning. Gene therapy approaches to human FHL remain in the distant future.

REFERENCES

1. Meeths M, Horne A, Sabel M, et al. Incidence and clinical presentation of primary hemophagocytic lymphohistiocytosis in Sweden. Pediatr Blood Cancer 2015;62: 346–52.

2. Ishii E, Ohga S, Imashuku S, et al. Nationwide survey of hemophagocytic lympho-histiocytosis in Japan. Int J Hematol 2007;86(1):58–65.
3. Farquhar JW, Claireaux AE. Familial haemophagocytic reticulosis. Arch Dis Child 1952;27(136):519–25.
4. Stepp SE, Dufourcq-Lagelouse R, Le Deist F, et al. Perforin gene defects in famil-ial hemophagocytic lymphohistiocytosis. Science 1999;286(5446):1957–9.
5. Ohadi M, Lalloz MR, Sham P, et al. Localization of a gene for familial hemopha-gocytic lymphohistiocytosis at chromosome 9q21.3-22 by homozygosity map-ping. Am J Hum Genet 1999;64(1):165–71.
6. Jordan MB, Filipovich AH. Hematopoietic cell transplantation for hemophagocytic lymphohistiocytosis: a journey of a thousand miles begins with a single (big) step. Bone Marrow Transplant 2008;42(7):433–7.
7. Trizzino A, zur Stadt U, Ueda I, et al. Genotype-phenotype study of familial hemopha-gocytic lymphohistiocytosis due to perforin mutations. J Med Genet 2007;45(1): 15–21.
8. Lee SM, Sumegi J, Villanueva J, et al. Patients of African ancestry with hemopha-gocytic lymphohistiocytosis share a common haplotype of PRF1 with a 50delT mutation. J Pediatr 2006;149(1):134–7.
9. Feldmann J, Callebaut I, Raposo G, et al. Munc13-4 is essential for cytolytic gran-ules fusion and is mutated in a form of familial hemophagocytic lymphohistiocy-tosis (FHL-3). Cell 2003;115(4):461–73.
10. Sieni E, Cetica V, Santoro A, et al. Genotype-phenotype study of familial haemo-phagocytic lymphohistiocytosis type 3. J Med Genet 2011;48(5):343–52.
11. Santoro A, Cannella S, Bossi G, et al. Novel Munc13-4 mutations in children and young adult patients with haemophagocytic lymphohistiocytosis. J Med Genet 2006;43(12):953–60.
12. zur Stadt U, Schmidt S, Kasper B, et al. Linkage of familial hemophagocytic lym-phohistiocytosis (FHL) type-4 to chromosome 6q24 and identification of muta-tions in syntaxin 11. Hum Mol Genet 2005;14(6):827–34.
13. Cote M, Ménager MM, Burgess A, et al. Munc18-2 deficiency causes familial he-mophagocytic lymphohistiocytosis type 5 and impairs cytotoxic granule exocy-tosis in patient NK cells. J Clin Invest 2009;119(12):3765–73.
14. Pagel J, Beutel K, Lehmberg K, et al. Distinct mutations in STXBP2 are associ-ated with variable clinical presentations in patients with familial hemophagocytic lymphohistiocytosis type 5 (FHL-5). Blood 2012;119(25):6016–24.
15. Nichols KE, Harkin DP, Levitz S, et al. Inactivating mutations in an SH2 domain-encoding gene in X-linked lymphoproliferative syndrome. Proc Natl Acad Sci U S A 1998;95(23):13765–70.
16. Rigaud S, Fondanèche MC, Lambert N, et al. XIAP deficiency in humans causes an X-linked lymphoproliferative syndrome. Nature 2006;444(7115):110–4.
17. Marsh RA, Madden L, Kitchen BJ, et al. XIAP deficiency: a unique primary im-munodeficiency best classified as X-linked familial hemophagocytic lymphohistio-cytosis and not as X-linked lymphoproliferative disease. Blood 2010;116(7): 1079–82.
18. Pachlopnik Schmid J, Canioni D, Moshous D, et al. Clinical similarities and differences of patients with X-linked lymphoproliferative syndrome type 1 (XLP-1/SAP deficiency) versus type 2 (XLP-2/XIAP deficiency). Blood 2011;117(5): 1522–9.
19. Menasche G, Pastural E, Feldmann J, et al. Mutations in RAB27A cause Griscelli syndrome associated with haemophagocytic syndrome. Nat Genet 2000;25(2): 173–6.

20. Meeths M, Bryceson YT, Rudd E, et al. Clinical presentation of Griscelli syndrome type 2 and spectrum of RAB27A mutations. Pediatr Blood Cancer 2010;54(4): 563–72.

21. Zhang K, Jordan MB, Marsh RA, et al. Hypomorphic mutations in PRF1, Munc13-4, and STXBP2 are associated with adult-onset familial HLH. Blood 2011;118(22): 5794–8.

22. Spessott WA, Sanmillan ML, McCormick ME, et al. Hemophagocytic lymphohistiocytosis caused by dominant-negative mutations in STXBP2 that inhibit SNARE-mediated membrane fusion. Blood 2015;125(10):1566–77.

23. Zhang K, Chandrakasan S, Chapman H, et al. Synergistic defects of different molecules in the cytotoxic pathway lead to clinical familial hemophagocytic lymphohistiocytosis. Blood 2014;124(8):1331–4.

24. Kaufman KM, Linghu B, Szustakowski JD, et al. Whole-exome sequencing reveals overlap between macrophage activation syndrome in systemic juvenile idiopathic arthritis and familial hemophagocytic lymphohistiocytosis. Arthritis Rheumatol 2014;66(12):3486–95.

25. Henter JI, Elinder G, Ost A. Diagnostic guidelines for hemophagocytic lymphohistiocytosis. The FHL Study Group of the Histiocyte Society. Semin Oncol 1991;18(1):29–33.

26. Henter JI, Horne A, Aricó M, et al. HLH-2004: diagnostic and therapeutic guidelines for hemophagocytic lymphohistiocytosis. Pediatr Blood Cancer 2007;48(2): 124–31.

27. Perez N, Virelizier JL, Arenzana-Seisdedos F, et al. Impaired natural killer activity in lymphohistiocytosis syndrome. J Pediatr 1984;104(4):569–73.

28. Ishii E, Ueda I, Shirakawa R, et al. Genetic subtypes of familial hemophagocytic lymphohistiocytosis: correlations with clinical features and cytotoxic T lymphocyte/natural killer cell functions. Blood 2005;105(9):3442–8.

29. Marcenaro S, Gallo F, Martini S, et al. Analysis of natural killer-cell function in familial hemophagocytic lymphohistiocytosis (FHL): defective CD107a surface expression heralds Munc13-4 defect and discriminates between genetic subtypes of the disease. Blood 2006;108(7):2316–23.

30. Bryceson YT, Pende D, Maul-Pavicic A, et al. A prospective evaluation of degranulation assays in the rapid diagnosis of familial hemophagocytic syndromes. Blood 2012;119(12):2754–63.

31. Janka GE. Familial hemophagocytic lymphohistiocytosis. Eur J Pediatr 1983; 140(3):221–30.

32. Ambruso DR, Hays T, Zwartjes WJ, et al. Successful treatment of lymphohistiocytic reticulosis with phagocytosis with epipodophyllotoxin VP 16-213. Cancer 1980;45(10):2516–20.

33. Johnson TS, Terrell CE, Millen SH, et al. Etoposide selectively ablates activated T cells to control the immunoregulatory disorder hemophagocytic lymphohistiocytosis. J Immunol 2014;192(1):84–91.

34. Henter JI, Samuelsson-Horne A, Aricò M, et al. Treatment of hemophagocytic lymphohistiocytosis with HLH-94 immunochemotherapy and bone marrow transplantation. Blood 2002;100(7):2367–73.

35. Mahlaoui N, Ouachée-Chardin M, de Saint Basile G, et al. Immunotherapy of familial hemophagocytic lymphohistiocytosis with antithymocyte globulins: a single-center retrospective report of 38 patients. Pediatrics 2007;120(3):e622–8.

36. Marsh RA, Allen CE, McClain KL, et al. Salvage therapy of refractory hemophagocytic lymphohistiocytosis with alemtuzumab. Pediatr Blood Cancer 2013; 60(1):101–9.

37. Horne A, Trottestam H, Aricò M, et al. Frequency and spectrum of central nervous system involvement in 193 children with haemophagocytic lymphohistiocytosis. Br J Haematol 2008;140(3):327–35.
38. Haddad E, Sulis ML, Jabado N, et al. Frequency and severity of central nervous system lesions in hemophagocytic lymphohistiocytosis. Blood 1997;89(3): 794–800.
39. Baker KS, Filipovich AH, Gross TG, et al. Unrelated donor hematopoietic cell transplantation for hemophagocytic lymphohistiocytosis. Bone Marrow Transplant 2008;42(3):175–80.
40. Fischer A, Cerf-Bensussan N, Blanche S, et al. Allogeneic bone marrow transplantation for erythrophagocytic lymphohistiocytosis. J Pediatr 1986;108(2): 267–70.
41. Trottestam H, Horne A, Aricò M, et al. Chemoimmunotherapy for hemophagocytic lymphohistiocytosis: long-term results of the HLH-94 treatment protocol. Blood 2011;118(17):4577–84.
42. Cooper N, Rao K, Gilmour K, et al. Stem cell transplantation with reduced-intensity conditioning for hemophagocytic lymphohistiocytosis. Blood 2006; 107(3):1233–6.
43. Marsh RA, Vaughn G, Kim MO, et al. Reduced-intensity conditioning significantly improves survival of patients with hemophagocytic lymphohistiocytosis undergoing allogeneic hematopoietic cell transplantation. Blood 2010;116(26):5824–31.

Hemophagocytic Lymphohistiocytosis in Adults

Meghan Campo, MD[b], Nancy Berliner, MD[a],*

KEYWORDS

- Hemophagocytic lymphohistiocytosis • Adults
- Acquired hemophagocytic lymphohistiocytosis • Treatment • Diagnosis

KEY POINTS

- Acquired hemophagocytic lymphohistiocytosis (HLH), though seen in the pediatric population, is the more common form of HLH in adults, often triggered by an underlying infection, malignancy, or rheumatologic condition.
- Acquired HLH is a highly morbid condition; if left untreated, patients survive for only a few months because of progressive multisystem organ failure.
- The treatment paradigm of adult HLH is largely based on the pediatric, HLH-1994 protocol. Further work is needed to refine the diagnostic criteria and treatment algorithm for the adult population.

INTRODUCTION

Hemophagocytic lymphohistiocytosis (HLH) is a rare but potentially fatal syndrome of pathologic immune dysregulation characterized by clinical signs and symptoms of extreme inflammation. The pathology of the condition centers on the activation and proliferation of uncontrolled macrophages and lymphocytes, culminating in an unrelenting cytokine storm and subsequent tissue infiltration and multiorgan system failure.

HLH can occur as a genetic or sporadic disorder and, though seen as an inherited condition affecting primarily a pediatric population, can occur at any age and be encountered in association with a variety of underlying diseases. Genetic HLH occurs in familial forms (fHLH), in which HLH is the primary and only manifestation, and in association with immune deficiencies such as Chédiak-Higashi syndrome, Griscelli syndrome, and X-linked lymphoproliferative syndrome, whereby secondary HLH occurs sporadically and is often a terminal phase of the disease. Acquired HLH,

[a] Division of Hematology, Brigham and Women's Hospital, Harvard Medical School, Mid-Campus 3, 75 Francis Street, Boston, MA 02115, USA; [b] Dana Farber Cancer Institue, Boston, MA, USA
* Corresponding author.
E-mail address: nberliner@partners.org

Hematol Oncol Clin N Am 29 (2015) 915–925
http://dx.doi.org/10.1016/j.hoc.2015.06.009
0889-8588/15/$ – see front matter © 2015 Elsevier Inc. All rights reserved.

though seen in the pediatric population, is the more common form of HLH in adults and is often triggered by an underlying infection, malignancy, or rheumatologic condition (**Box 1**). Clinically the syndrome, whether genetic or acquired, is characterized by fever, hepatosplenomegaly, cytopenias, and the finding of activated macrophages in hematopoietic organs, often resulting in multiorgan system failure and death. Therapy centers on the suppression of this hyperinflammatory state, focusing on the destruction of cytotoxic T lymphocytes and macrophages with cytotoxic, immunosuppressive therapy and treatment of any existing HLH triggers.

ACQUIRED HEMOPHAGOCYTIC LYMPHOHISTIOCYTOSIS

Acquired HLH can present at any age, although it is more typically encountered in the adult population with a mean age at diagnosis of 48 to 50 years old.[1,2] It is associated with a wide variety of conditions including infection, malignancy, autoimmune disorders, and immunosuppression. These entities have been linked to the development of HLH in the literature; however, there are also case reports of lesser described triggers including medications, pregnancy, and post-hematologic and solid organ transplantation.

The clinical presentation of acquired HLH is similar to the familial form, and the diagnostic criteria remain the same. However, as the criteria for diagnosis were developed in the context of pediatric patients, there is considerable interest in adapting the diagnostic criteria to improve the diagnosis of HLH in adults. Genetic testing in these patients reveals a subset that displays heterozygous mutations and polymorphisms in the known fHLH genes (**Table 1**). In one study of adult patients who met the criteria for HLH, missense and splice-site sequence variants in *PRF1*, *MUNC13-4*, and *STXBP2* were present in 14% of patients, and the A91V-PRF1 genotype was found in 4.8%.[3] Hypomorphic alleles for fHLH genes are implicated in approximately 15% of acquired HLH. However, to date there are no data to indicate whether the prognosis of patients who possess these defects differs from those in whom such polymorphisms are not identified.[3]

Box 1
Conditions associated with HLH

Genetic

1. Familial
   - Known genetic defects: *PRF1, MUNC13-4, STX1, STXBP2*
   - Unknown genetic defects

2. Immune deficiency syndromes
   - Chédiak-Higashi syndrome, Griscelli syndrome, X-linked lymphoproliferative syndrome: *LYST, RAB27α*

Acquired

1. Infections
   - Viral, bacterial, fungal

2. Malignancy

3. Autoimmune conditions

4. Others: posttransplantation, pregnancy, drug-induced

Table 1 HLH subtypes and their known genetic defects		
HLH Subtype	**Genetic Defect**	**Resulting Defect**
FHL1	9q21.3-locus 6	Unknown
FHL2	*PRF1*	Vesicle content
FHL3	*UNC13D*	Defective cytolytic granule exocytosis
FHL4	*STX18B*	Defective intracellular transport
FHL5	*UNC18B*	Defective membrane fusion

Data from Tothova Z, Berliner N. Hemophagocytic syndrome and critical illness: new insights into diagnosis and management. J Intensive Care Med 2014 Jan 8. [Epub ahead of print].

Infection

Viral infection, either as a primary infection or reactivation in an immunosuppressed host, is a frequent trigger of acquired HLH. In a large study of 96 adult patients from Taiwan with HLH, 30 were associated with infection.[4] The most common types of infection were viral (41%), mycobacterial (23%), bacterial (23%), and fungal (13%). The Epstein-Barr virus (EBV) is the most common viral pathogen linked to the development of HLH. EBV is postulated to cause a clonal proliferation and hyperactivation of EBV-infected T cells in patients with EBV-associated HLH. Other viral pathogens linked to the disorder include cytomegalovirus, parvovirus, herpes simplex virus, norovirus, varicella zoster virus, measles virus, human herpes virus 8, H1N1 influenza virus, and human immunodeficiency virus (HIV). In one retrospective analysis of 162 patients with HLH, approximately 25% were found to have an infectious trigger, with approximately half of these cases thought to be secondary to HIV.[2] Although less commonly reported, HLH may also occur in the setting of infections caused by bacteria (*Mycobacterium tuberculosis*, *Ricksettsia*, *Escherichia coli*), parasites (*Leishmania*), and fungi (*Histoplasma*).

Malignancy

The development of HLH in individuals with an underlying malignancy has been clearly described. The hematologic malignancies, specifically lymphoma, are the most common cause of malignancy-associated HLH. Among lymphomas, T-cell lymphoproliferative disorders, such as anaplastic large cell lymphoma and natural killer (NK) cell lymphoma, are the most frequently linked to HLH. A recent survey of adult patients with HLH reported that more than half (52%) were associated with malignancies. Of these cases, approximately 59% were associated with T-cell lymphoma and 19% were linked to diffuse large B-cell lymphoma.[5] Data are limited as to whether the malignancy itself is causative of HLH or whether the malignancy places the patient at increased risk of infection that ultimately triggers the syndrome.

Autoimmune Conditions, Macrophage Activation Syndrome

Several autoimmune conditions are known precipitants of HLH including systemic lupus erythematosus (SLE), mixed connective tissue disorder, dermatomyositis, systemic sclerosis, and Kikuchi disease. HLH may develop at any time during the course of a rheumatologic disorder, on presentation, during therapy, or at time of flare.[6] The specific term macrophage activation syndrome (MAS) is typically used when a hemophagocytic syndrome develops in children with juvenile idiopathic arthritis and other rheumatologic conditions, but it has also been documented as a syndrome in adults, the limited data for which suggest that it is seen most frequently in association with adult-onset Still disease, SLE, and various vasculitic syndromes. The primary clinical manifestations of adult-onset MAS are identical to those in pediatric patients and include fever, lymphadenopathy, hepatosplenomegaly, and liver function test (LFT) derangements. In addition to similar clinical manifestations, MAS and HLH also share genetic similarities. Polymorphisms and heterozygous mutations in *PRF1* and *UNC13D* have been identified in MAS patients, most of whom also have decreased NK function, elevated soluble CD25 (sCD25), and elevated soluble CD163 (sCD163).[7]

Diagnosis

The diagnosis of acquired HLH, especially in adults, is often difficult, and may frequently not be considered or confirmed before a patient's death. The primary problem is the lack of a specific disease marker, as the clinical picture is often nonspecific and mimics alternative infectious or malignant conditions. Many of the initial, nonspecific tests that are helpful in evaluating HLH (complete blood count, coagulation studies, and LFTs) are completed in the evaluation of an unexplained febrile illness. Additional markers, including serum ferritin, triglycerides, and screening immunologic studies, are ordered when suspicion for HLH mounts.

Although the significance of the results remains to be determined, the author recommends that mutation analysis be requested for all adult cases of confirmed or suspected HLH at some time during their course, with analysis of the known fHLH mutations (*PRF1*, *UNC13D*, *STX11*, and *UNC18B*), as a subset will possess heterozygous mutations and polymorphisms in the known fHLH genes. That said, negative results will be found in most of the adult population. As the presence or absence of a mutation does not alter treatment, appropriate therapy should not be delayed while awaiting results, and in fact testing need not be done at the time of initial evaluation. However, the presence of an fHLH mutation may provide guidance in decisions regarding ongoing therapy or transplantation for patients who achieve remission with initial HLH therapy. It must be stressed that the clinical importance of finding hypomorphic fHLH alleles remains to be established in the adult population, but whether such mutations predict a course that is different from that in patients without mutations should become clearer as the disease becomes better recognized and testing becomes more universal. The Histiocyte Society developed a set of diagnostic criteria in 1994 to help clinicians identify pediatric patients with both familial and acquired HLH on clinical and laboratory grounds. These criteria were later refined in 2004 (**Box 2**) to include decreased NK-cell function and elevated sCD25 or serum-soluble interleukin-2 receptor (sIL-2R) levels. It should be noted that although these recently added markers (NK function, sIL-2R) are helpful in establishing a diagnosis, testing often requires sending samples to specialized laboratories, and these results are not always available to help with a timely diagnosis. It should also be recognized that these criteria were developed for the diagnosis of pediatric patients and may not be best suited to making the diagnosis of HLH in adults.

Clinical Manifestations

Adult HLH often presents as a febrile illness with multiorgan involvement that mimics common viral and bacterial infections. Patients typically present with high, prolonged fever and findings on physical examination of hepatomegaly, splenomegaly, and lymphadenopathy. Laboratory evaluation reveals the presence of LFT abnormalities, elevated ferritin, and cytopenias, most commonly anemia and thrombocytopenia. With few exceptions, the clinical manifestations are similar regardless of whether an underlying genetic defect is present and identified.

> **Box 2**
> **Diagnostic criteria for the diagnosis of HLH**
>
> *The diagnosis of HLH can be established if A or B is fulfilled*
>
> A. A molecular diagnosis consistent with HLH
>
> - Pathologic mutations of *PRF1, UNC13D, STXBP1, RAB27A, STX11, SH2D1A,* or *XIAP*
>
> B. Five of the following clinical criteria
>
> - Fever
>
> - Splenomegaly
>
> - Peripheral cytopenias (affecting at least 2 of 3 cell lineages)
>
> - Hypertriglyceridemia (fasting, >3 mmol/L) and/or hypofibrinogenemia (<1.5 g/dL)
>
> - Hemophagocytosis in bone marrow, spleen, lymph nodes, or liver
>
> - Ferritin greater than 500 μg/L
>
> - Low or absent natural killer cell activity
>
> - Increased soluble CD25 concentration (α chain of soluble interleukin-2 receptor) greater than 2400 U/mL
>
> *Data from* Henter JI, Horne A, Arico M, et al. HLH-2004: diagnostic and therapeutic guidelines for hemophagocytic lymphohistiocytosis. Pediatr Blood Cancer 2007;48:124–31.

Neurologic Manifestations

Neurologic manifestations are variable in presentation, and include focal neurologic deficits, seizure, encephalopathy, coma, and sensory and motor peripheral neuropathy resulting from myelin destruction by macrophages.[7] Approximately one-third of all patients with HLH will develop some degree of neurologic dysfunction during the course of their disease. The variability in presentation is similar to that found in laboratory and imaging findings, which makes the diagnosis of central nervous system (CNS) involvement difficult. In children with HLH, approximately 50% will have abnormalities of the cerebrospinal fluid (CSF), with most demonstrating a pleocytosis.[8] MRI of the brain of these same patients may show discrete lesions, leptomeningeal enhancement, and hypodense or necrotic areas, or may be completely normal.[9] However, in adult patients these laboratory and imaging findings are thought to be much less prevalent and have been restricted to case reports.[10] Regardless of the exact clinical manifestation in both the pediatric and adult population, the presence of neurologic involvement is thought to be a poor prognostic marker.[8,11]

Dermatologic Manifestations

Patients with adult HLH may have a wide array of cutaneous findings including generalized erythroderma, generalized maculopapular rash, petechiae, and purpura. Biopsies have shown that rashes may correlate with lymphocytic infiltration and frank hemophagocytosis. Close attention should be paid to those with subcutaneous panniculitic–like nodules attributable to the association with an underlying T-cell lymphoma.[1] These variable dermatologic manifestations are thought to be rare, although dermatologists have suggested that maculopapular rashes are fairly common.[12,13]

Laboratory Findings

Characteristic laboratory findings in all patients with HLH include liver function abnormalities, elevated ferritin, coagulopathy, hypertriglyceridemia, and cytopenias affecting at least 2 lineages in the peripheral blood. These abnormalities are thought to be driven in large part by the hypercytokinemia that pervades this disorder.

Elevated ferritin

Ferritin has proved to be a valuable diagnostic and prognostic marker in cases of pediatric HLH. In pediatric populations, a ferritin greater than 10,000 mg/dL is 90% sensitive and 96% specific for a diagnosis of HLH.[14] However, although virtually all adults with HLH meet the diagnostic criteria of a ferritin count greater than 500 mg/dL, the sensitivity and specificity of this marker in the adult population is much less impressive. A study examining the correlation between HLH and hyper-ferritinemia in adult hospitalized patients with extremely high ferritin levels (>50,000 mg/dL) was recently reported. The specificity of the ferritin level was low in this group of adults, with a confirmed HLH diagnosed in only 19 of 111 individuals. Extreme elevations of ferritin were more typically seen with hepatocellular insult, renal failure, infections, and hematologic malignancies.[15] Consequently, although the negative predictive value of a normal serum ferritin is high, there is no level of ferritin that has high positive predictive value in diagnosing HLH.

Hemophagocytosis

Hemophagocytosis is defined by phagocytosis by histiocytes of erythrocytes, leukocytes, platelets, and their precursors in bone marrow and other tissues. In the pediatric literature the reported incidence of hemophagocytosis detected on biopsy ranges from 25% to 100%.[7] This phenomenon, though semantically linked to HLH, is neither sensitive nor specific for the diagnosis, and is considered one of the less important diagnostic criteria even in cases of fHLH. More frequently, hemophagocytosis is induced by more common events such as infection, autoimmune conditions, and blood transfusions.[7]

In HLH, histologic examination of any involved organs may show infiltration by histiocytes and lymphocytes, with hemophagocytosis.[11,16] Evidence of hemophagocytosis at any biopsy site fulfills diagnostic criteria; however, bone marrow aspiration[11] is often the diagnostic modality of choice. Spleen biopsy has inherent complications, and liver biopsy is often uninformative because it often reveals a hepatitis-like lymphocytic infiltration rather than frank hemophagocytosis. Repeat bone marrow biopsy is often needed, as in most cases hemophagocytosis may not be observed in the initial bone marrow aspirate but will become evident on follow-up evaluation.

Liver function abnormality and coagulopathy

Though not part of the HLH-2004 diagnostic criteria, liver inflammation is almost always evident in adult patients with newly diagnosed HLH. Abnormalities range from mild transaminitis or cholestasis to fulminant hepatic failure. The prevalence of hepatic dysfunction is so high that normal LFTs should bring into question the diagnosis of HLH. Liver biopsy, if performed, is likely to show infiltration of lymphocytes into the portal tracts similar to that seen in chronic persistent hepatitis.[16] Bleeding complications are common in this condition and are seen in up to 60% of patients.[1] Hemorrhage may reflect a variety of factors, including coagulopathy from liver dysfunction, thrombocytopenia from bone marrow failure, or platelet function defects associated with an underlying genetic defect in platelet granules.[7]

Soluble CD163

CD163, a receptor for hemoglobin-haptoglobin complexes and a marker of macrophage activation, is of growing interest. Although increased plasma levels of sCD163 are seen in malignancy, autoimmune conditions, and infection, levels are considerably higher in patients with HLH.[17] Though not specific for this disorder, in combination with additional clinical and laboratory findings suggestive of HLH, it can assist clinicians in establishing a diagnosis.

Depressed natural killer function

Demonstration of very low NK function can support a diagnosis of HLH. NK-cell activity can be measured by several modalities, including the ^{51}Cr release assay. In this assay, chromium-labeled NK cells are stimulated to degranulate. Release of the radionuclide is expected to be reduced or absent in HLH. The reported sensitivity of these tests approaches 100%. One study looking at 13 patients with adult HLH noted lower NK-cell activity in patients with confirmed HLH compared with controls.[18] However, studies demonstrate that even in genetically confirmed cases of fHLH, NK function may be normal, suggesting that preserved NK function does not preclude the diagnosis.[17,19] Furthermore, in most studies of adult HLH the NK function is seldom tested. For example, in the 62 patients who met the HLH-2004 diagnostic criteria in one study, only 5 had NK function tested, 3 of whom (60%) had depressed or absent NK function.[5]

Elevated serum-soluble interleukin-2 receptor

Measurement of the α chain of the soluble interleukin (IL)-2 receptor (sCD25), reflecting the degree of activation of T cells, can aid in confirming a diagnosis of HLH. Although recent studies have illustrated that levels of sIL-2Rα vary with age, very high levels are almost never seen outside HLH (Fill ASH, Weitzman ASH). Of note, recent studies have investigated sIL-2R/ferritin ratio as a marker to diagnose lymphoma-associated hemophagocytic syndrome (LAHS), which is a major subtype of adult-onset HLH. One study found that the mean sIL-2R levels were significantly higher in the LAHS group, whereas the ferritin levels were higher in the benign disease–associated HLH group. Consequently, the mean serum sIL-2R/ferritin ratio of patients with LAHS was markedly higher than that of patients with benign disease–associated HLH, thus demonstrating that the serum sIL-2R/ferritin ratio is a useful marker for diagnosing LAHS.[20]

Prognosis

The pediatric HLH-94 protocol yielded important early insights into HLH prognosis in children. In that study, the presence of elevated ferritin (>2000 µg/L), elevated bilirubin, and abnormal CSF findings correlated with increased mortality. Work is under way to identify prognostic factors in adult HLH, and although there has been no large scale prospective analysis there are several published retrospective case reviews. In adult HLH, prognosis seems to be negatively affected by the presence of underlying malignancy, certain laboratory abnormalities, and diagnosis at an older age.[21] Malignancy-associated HLH, specifically in the setting of T-cell lymphoma, fares poorly when compared with those cases driven by infectious or rheumatologic conditions,[5] with case series noting a median overall survival of 1 month versus 46 months for those with nonmalignant HLH.[22] In EBV-associated HLH, a high viral DNA load is associated with poor outcomes. Other laboratory findings including hypoalbuminemia, thrombocytopenia, and hyperferritinemia (>50,000 µg/L) have been shown to correlate with increased mortality in adult patients.[5,22,23]

Treatment

Acquired HLH is a highly morbid condition, and if left untreated patients survive for only a few months owing to progressive multisystem organ failure, with overall mortality ranging from to 41% to 75%.[1,24] However, those patients with confirmed infectious or autoimmune triggers tend to have better outcomes, with mortality ranging from 8% to 24%.[25] Because of the high morbidity and mortality of the disorder, an aggressive therapeutic approach with rapid treatment of HLH is necessary, and therapy should not be delayed while awaiting molecular studies or other ancillary tests such as sCD25. In general, treatment entails the suppression of an overactive immune system and, in cases where a trigger is identified, focused therapy on the underlying cause. The current treatment of adult or acquired HLH is based on the pediatric HLH-94/-2004 protocols.

The first international treatment protocol for HLH, primarily designed to treat pediatric disease, was initiated by the Histiocyte Society in 1994.[26] This regimen entails an 8-week induction course of dexamethasone, etoposide, and intrathecal methotrexate. The principal goal of induction therapy is to suppress the overwhelming inflammatory process that drives HLH. Patients who complete the 8-week induction course and recover normal immune function and have no identified HLH-associated gene defects may stop therapy. If disease worsens during induction therapy while etoposide and dexamethasone are being tapered, indicated by progressive laboratory or clinical derangements, the doses can be escalated to full dose. Those who require additional therapy because of persistent disease are transitioned to continuation therapy, which in pediatrics is usually viewed as a bridge to hematopoietic cell transplantation (HCT). Continuation according to HLH-94 consists of pulses of dexamethasone and etoposide with the addition of cyclosporine in patients who are hemodynamically stable and have adequate liver and kidney function. In current practice, tacrolimus is often substituted for cyclosporine in adults, as it leads to less nephrotoxicity. Continuation therapy followed by HCT is recommended in pediatric patients with refractory disease and those with a high risk of relapse, including those with CNS involvement, persistent NK-cell dysfunction, documented homozygous or compound heterozygous HLH gene mutations, recurrent or progressive disease despite intensive therapy, and hematologic malignancy that cannot be cured otherwise.[7] The therapeutic indications for stem cell transplantation remain to be established for adults, but it is usually recommended for those who relapse or fail to achieve remission. It is also usually recommended for those who are found to have fHLH-related mutations (usually posited to be hypomorphic alleles), despite the lack of evidence that the latter group have a higher risk of recurrence.

The same group responsible for the HLH-94 protocol refined their treatment paradigm in 2004. The HLH-2004 protocol includes cyclosporine in the induction regimen and additionally adds hydrocortisone to intrathecal methotrexate for treatment of CNS disease.[27] The results of the treatment changes in the HLH-2004 protocol are not yet known. Without the final interpretation of HLH-2004 available, the risks and benefits of adding cyclosporine to the induction phase remain unconfirmed, and most clinicians continue to treat according to the protocol set forth by HLH-94.

Refractory/Recurrent Disease

After completion of induction therapy, a subset of patients demonstrates persistent disease or relapse shortly thereafter, and salvage therapy becomes necessary. In the pediatric literature, relapse typically occurs within a year of the initial acute illness, and these patients are more likely to harbor an HLH gene mutation than their counterparts who maintain remission.[7] Patients, both pediatric and adult, who have initially achieved disease remission with the HLH-94 protocol are often retreated with the same regimen. Studies have looked at the incorporation of alternative agents to etoposide and dexamethasone, such as alemtuzumab. A monoclonal antibody to the CD52 protein expressed on the surface of mature T cells and possibly NK cells, alemtuzumab has been administered in patients with refractory disease. In a study of 22 pediatric and adult patients treated with alemtuzumab, a partial response was seen in 86%, and 77% were able to ultimately undergo HCT.[28]

Treatment of Specific Populations

Treatment of the clinically stable patient

Patients who are stable and have an identifiable condition responsible for triggering HLH, such as an underlying infection, may respond to treatment of the triggering condition alone. However, deterioration during the search for, or therapy for, the underlying condition is an indication to start HLH-specific therapy immediately.

Infectious trigger

Infections are a major trigger for adult HLH, and appropriately targeted antimicrobial and antiviral therapy is a cornerstone of management. Patients who are clinically stable and respond within a few days to treatment of an identified infection (bacterial, viral, fungal) may be able to avoid HLH-specific chemotherapy. However, initiation of HLH-specific therapy for severely ill patients should not be delayed while awaiting resolution of an identified infection.

Specifically for EBV-triggered cases of HLH, etoposide is a crucial therapeutic agent that must be added before disease response is achieved. The importance of etoposide is demonstrated in one large Japanese series involving patients with EBV HLH where survival was significantly improved if etoposide was initiated early and if at least 4 doses of etoposide were administered.[25] Rituximab has also demonstrated therapeutic benefit in EBV HLH as an adjunct to anti-HLH therapy. EBV largely resides in B lymphocytes, which can be rapidly depleted using the monoclonal antibody directed against the CD20 antigen on B lymphocytes. Depletion of B cells, which serve as a reservoir for EBV, is thought to improve survival by not only eradicating an HLH reservoir but also preventing relapse. The efficacy of rituximab in the treatment of HLH was investigated in 42 patients who were treated with rituximab-containing regimens. These patients, on average, received 3 rituximab infusions at a median dose of 375 mg/m^2, along with steroids, etoposide, and/or cyclosporine. Overall the therapy was well tolerated and resulted in clinical improvements in 43% of the patients, with most demonstrating reduced EBV viral loads.[29] However, as EBV also infects non–B-cell populations (T and NK cells) in patients with HLH, monotherapy with rituximab is not thought to be effective in eradicating HLH, and therefore must be used in concert with additional agents such as etoposide and dexamethasone.

Rheumatologic trigger

Treatment of a patient with an underlying rheumatologic condition centers on successful management of the underlying rheumatologic entity, which typically involves high-dose immunosuppressive agents. In cases of MAS, high-dose immunosuppression is the initial treatment of choice. However, in cases proven to be steroid refractory, cyclosporine has been found to be effective.[30] In addition to immunosuppression, investigators are studying the effects of several monoclonal antibodies in the treatment of MAS. Recent studies of patients with adult-onset Still disease complicated by MAS have evaluated the efficacy of the IL-1 receptor antagonist anakinra and the IL-6 receptor tocilizumab.[31,32] Although small case reports have been promising, there is concern that the inhibition of a single cytokine by a biological response modifier may be of limited efficacy for the treatment of the cytokine storm that is present in MAS. Confirmation of the efficacy of these agents awaits larger trials.

Oncologic trigger
For patients with disease thought to be driven by a hematologic malignancy, recommendations are made to treat with HLH-specific therapy, followed by appropriate chemotherapy for the malignancy with the caveat that HCT is often required.

FUTURE DIRECTIONS

HLH, though once considered a predominantly pediatric condition, is increasingly recognized in the adult population. Like its pediatric counterpart, adult HLH is a highly morbid condition that is almost universally fatal if unrecognized or untreated. At present there is little evidence to guide the evaluation, diagnosis, and treatment of HLH in the adult population. Further work is needed to discover clinically useful markers of the disease that can refine the current diagnostic criteria. With regard to treatment, further elucidation of genetic alterations and predisposing medical conditions linked to HLH should increase the understanding of the underlying pathogenesis, and lead to the development and implementation of more disease-specific therapies and improved outcomes in adults with HLH.

REFERENCES

1. Ramos-Casals M, Brito-Zeron P, Lopez-Guillermo A, et al. Adult haemophagocytic syndrome. Lancet 2014;383:1503–16.
2. Riviere S, Galicier L, Coppo P, et al. Reactive hemophagocytic syndrome in adults: a retrospective analysis of 162 patients. Am J Med 2014;127:1118–25.
3. Zhang K, Jordan MB, Marsh RA, et al. Hypomorphic mutations in PRF1, MUNC13-4, and STXBP2 are associated with adult-onset familial HLH. Blood 2011;118:5794–8.
4. Tseng YT, Sheng WH, Lin BH, et al. Causes, clinical symptoms, and outcomes of infectious diseases associated with hemophagocytic lymphohistiocytosis in Taiwanese adults. J Microbiol Immunol Infect 2011;44:191–7.
5. Parikh SA, Kapoor P, Letendre L, et al. Prognostic factors and outcomes of adults with hemophagocytic lymphohistiocytosis. Mayo Clin Proc 2014;89:484–92.
6. Fukaya S, Yasuda S, Hashimoto T, et al. Clinical features of haemophagocytic syndrome in patients with systemic autoimmune diseases: analysis of 30 cases. Rheumatology 2008;47:1686–91.
7. Jordan MB, Allen CE, Weitzman S, et al. How I treat hemophagocytic lymphohistiocytosis. Blood 2011;118:4041–52.
8. Haddad E, Sulis ML, Jabado N, et al. Frequency and severity of central nervous system lesions in hemophagocytic lymphohistiocytosis. Blood 1997;89:794–800.
9. Henter JI, Nennesmo I. Neuropathologic findings and neurologic symptoms in twenty-three children with hemophagocytic lymphohistiocytosis. J Pediatr 1997;130:358–65.
10. Clementi R, Emmi L, Maccario R, et al. Adult onset and atypical presentation of hemophagocytic lymphohistiocytosis in siblings carrying PRF1 mutations. Blood 2002;100:2266–7.
11. Akima M, Sumi SM. Neuropathology of familial erythrophagocytic lymphohistiocytosis: six cases and review of the literature. Hum Pathol 1984;15:161–8.
12. Morrell DS, Pepping MA, Scott JP, et al. Cutaneous manifestations of hemophagocytic lymphohistiocytosis. Arch Dermatol 2002;138:1208–12.
13. Fardet L, Galicier L, Vignon-Pennamen MD, et al. Frequency, clinical features and prognosis of cutaneous manifestations in adult patients with reactive haemophagocytic syndrome. Br J Dermatol 2010;162:547–53.

14. Allen CE, Yu X, Kozinetz CA, et al. Highly elevated ferritin levels and the diagnosis of hemophagocytic lymphohistiocytosis. Pediatr Blood Cancer 2008;50:1227–35.
15. Schram AM, Campigotto F, Mullally A, et al. Marked hyperferritinemia does not predict for HLH in the adult population. Blood 2015;125:1548–52.
16. Ost A, Nilsson-Ardnor S, Henter JI. Autopsy findings in 27 children with haemo-phagocytic lymphohistiocytosis. Histopathology 1998;32:310–6.
17. Weitzman S. Approach to hemophagocytic syndromes. Hematology Am Soc Hematol Educ Program 2011;2011:178–83.
18. Chung HJ, Park CJ, Lim JH, et al. Establishment of a reference interval for natural killer cell activity through flow cytometry and its clinical application in the diag-nosis of hemophagocytic lymphohistiocytosis. Int J Lab Hematol 2010;32: 239–47.
19. Filipovich AH. Hemophagocytic lymphohistiocytosis (HLH) and related disorders. Hematology Am Soc Hematol Educ Program 2009;127–31.
20. Tsuji T, Hirano T, Yamasaki H, et al. A high sIL-2R/ferritin ratio is a useful marker for the diagnosis of lymphoma-associated hemophagocytic syndrome. Ann Hematol 2014;93:821–6.
21. Kaito K, Kobayashi M, Katayama T, et al. Prognostic factors of hemophagocytic syndrome in adults: analysis of 34 cases. Eur J Haematol 1997;59:247–53.
22. Otrock ZK, Eby CS. Clinical characteristics, prognostic factors, and outcomes of adult patients with hemophagocytic lymphohistiocytosis. Am J Hematol 2015;90: 220–4.
23. Arca M, Fardet L, Galicier L, et al. Prognostic factors of early death in a cohort of 162 adult haemophagocytic syndrome: impact of triggering disease and early treatment with etoposide. Br J Haematol 2015;168:63–8.
24. Li J, Wang Q, Zheng W, et al. Hemophagocytic lymphohistiocytosis: clinical analysis of 103 adult patients. Medicine 2014;93:100–5.
25. Imashuku S. Treatment of Epstein-Barr virus-related hemophagocytic lymphohis-tiocytosis (EBV-HLH); update 2010. J Pediatr Hematol Oncol 2011;33:35–9.
26. Trottestam H, Horne A, Arico M, et al. Chemoimmunotherapy for hemophagocytic lymphohistiocytosis: long-term results of the HLH-94 treatment protocol. Blood 2011;118:4577–84.
27. Henter JI, Horne A, Arico M, et al. HLH-2004: diagnostic and therapeutic guide-lines for hemophagocytic lymphohistiocytosis. Pediatr Blood Cancer 2007;48: 124–31.
28. Marsh RA, Allen CE, McClain KL, et al. Salvage therapy of refractory hemopha-gocytic lymphohistiocytosis with alemtuzumab. Pediatr Blood Cancer 2013;60: 101–9.
29. Chellapandian D, Das R, Zelley K, et al. Treatment of Epstein Barr virus-induced haemophagocytic lymphohistiocytosis with rituximab-containing chemo-immuno-therapeutic regimens. Br J Haematol 2013;162:376–82.
30. Ravelli A. Macrophage activation syndrome. Curr Opin Rheumatol 2002;14: 548–52.
31. Durand M, Troyanov Y, Laflamme P, et al. Macrophage activation syndrome treated with anakinra. J Rheumatol 2010;37:879–80.
32. Sakai R, Nagasawa H, Nishi E, et al. Successful treatment of adult-onset Still's disease with tocilizumab monotherapy: two case reports and literature review. Clin Rheumatol 2012;31:569–74.

Macrophage Activation Syndrome

Angelo Ravelli, MD[a],*, Sergio Davì, MD[b], Francesca Minoia, MD[b], Alberto Martini[c], Randy Q. Cron, MD, PhD[d]

KEYWORDS

- Macrophage activation syndrome • Systemic juvenile idiopathic arthritis
- Hemophagocytic lymphohistiocytosis • Hemophagocytic syndrome
- Proinflammatory cytokines • Interleukin-1 inhibitors

KEY POINTS

- Macrophage activation syndrome (MAS) is a potentially life-threatening complication of rheumatic disorders, particularly systemic juvenile idiopathic arthritis.
- Although the pathophysiology of MAS is unclear, it is characterized by a dysfunctional immune response that is similar to that seen in other forms of hemophagocytic lymphohistiocytosis.
- Because MAS may pursue a rapidly fatal course, prompt recognition of its clinical and laboratory features and immediate therapeutic intervention are imperative.
- Recently, a set of classification criteria for MAS complicating systemic juvenile idiopathic arthritis has been developed through a multinational collaborative effort.
- The role of cytokine inhibitors in the management of MAS deserves further studies, although recent data about interleukin-1 antagonists are promising.

INTRODUCTION

The term macrophage activation syndrome (MAS) refers to a potentially life-threatening complication of rheumatic disorders that is seen most commonly in systemic juvenile idiopathic arthritis (sJIA)[1,2] and in its adult equivalent, adult-onset Still

Conflicts of interest: The authors declare no commercial or financial conflict of interest.
Funding: No funding source was available for this work.
[a] Department of Neuroscience, Rehabilitation, Ophthalmology, Genetics, Maternal and Child Health, Head, Center of Rheumatology, University of Genoa and G. Gaslini Institute, via G. Gaslini 5, Genoa 16147, Italy; [b] Second Pediatric Division and Rheumatology, G. Gaslini Institute, via G. Gaslini 5, Genoa 16147, Italy; [c] Department of Pediatrics and Second Pediatric Division and Rheumatology, University of Genoa and G. Gaslini Institute, via G. Gaslini 5, Genoa 16147, Italy; [d] Director, Division of Pediatric Rheumatology, Children's Hospital of Alabama and University of Alabama at Birmingham, Children's Park Place, Ste. 210 1601 4th Avenue South Birmingham, AL 35233, USA
* Corresponding author.
E-mail address: angeloravelli@ospedale-gaslini.ge.it

disease,[3] although it is encountered with increasing frequency in systemic lupus erythematosus of either childhood or adult onset[4,5] and Kawasaki disease.[6] In spite of recent reports in periodic fever syndromes,[7,8] the occurrence of MAS in other autoinflammatory diseases is rare.

This article summarizes the characteristics of MAS occurring in the context of sJIA and discusses the recent advances in classification systems and management.

HISTORY, NOMENCLATURE, AND CLASSIFICATION

The first description of this condition dates back to 1985, when Hadchouel and colleagues[9] reported a clinical syndrome of acute hemorrhagic, hepatic, and neurologic abnormalities in patients with sJIA. The term MAS was proposed in 1993 by the same group of investigators, who found evidence of activation of the monocyte-macrophage system in patients with the syndrome and noticed that its clinical features were very similar to those observed in hemophagocytic lymphohistiocytosis (HLH).[10] The recognition that MAS belongs to the spectrum of HLH has subsequently led to a proposal to rename it according to the contemporary classifications of HLH[11] and to classify it among the secondary, or acquired, forms of HLH.[12,13]

EPIDEMIOLOGY

The incidence of MAS in sJIA is unknown. It is estimated that around 10% of children with this disease develop overt MAS, but recent data suggest that the syndrome may occur subclinically or in mild form in another 30% to 40% of cases.[14,15] In a recent multinational study of 362 patients, MAS occurred more frequently in girls, with a female/male ratio of 6:4.[16] This slight female predominance contrasts with the 1:1 sex ratio typical of sJIA. The median time interval between the onset of sJIA and the occurrence of MAS was 4 months, and MAS was diagnosed simultaneously with sJIA in 22% of the patients. The demographic, clinical, laboratory, and histopathologic features of MAS were overall comparable among patients seen in different geographic areas.[17]

PATHOGENESIS

An in-depth discussion of the pathogenesis of MAS is beyond the scope of this article, and has been covered recently elsewhere.[18–20] However, a few developments are worth noting. The starting point for most pathogenetic studies is the notion that MAS is characterized by a dysfunctional immune response that is similar to that seen in other forms of HLH. The prototype of these is familial HLH (FHLH), which is a constellation of rare autosomal recessive immune disorders resulting from homozygous deficiency in cytolytic pathway proteins.[12,13,21] In FHLH, the uncontrolled expansion of T cells and macrophages has been attributed to diminished natural killer (NK) cell and cytotoxic T cell function,[12,13,21,22] caused by mutations in particular genes whose products are involved in the perforin-mediated cytolytic pathway.[23–26] These mutations cause profound impairment of cytotoxic function, which, through mechanisms that have not yet been fully elucidated, leads to an exaggerated expansion and activation of cytotoxic cells with hypersecretion of proinflammatory cytokines, which ultimately results in hematologic alterations and organ damage.[27] Recent evidence suggests that defects in killing leads to prolonged interaction between the cluster of differentiation 8 (CD8) T cell or NK cell and the infected target cell, resulting in a proinflammatory cytokine storm.[28]

Although the pathophysiology of MAS is less clear, it probably involves related pathogenic pathways.[29,30] It has recently been shown that, as in FHLH, patients with MAS may have functional abnormalities of the exosome degranulation pathway involved in perforin-mediated cytolysis.[31–33] Furthermore, several studies suggest the presence of some genetic overlap between MAS and FHLH. The same biallelic mutations in the MUNC13-4 gene reported in FHLH have been identified in some patients with sJIA with MAS.[34,35] Some of these mutations have been suggested to function as monoallelic dominant negative mutations disrupting cytolyisis.[35,36] Interferon regulatory factor 5 (IRF5) gene polymorphisms were also found to be risk factors for MAS in patients with sJIA.[37] Whole-exome sequencing has led to the discovery of rare protein-altering variants in known HLH-associated genes as well as in new candidate genes.[38]

In spite of the compelling evidence for a pathogenetic role of defects in cytotoxic cell function in FHLH, in many instances of MAS no such defects have been identified, or they have been found to have only variable penetrance. This finding has prompted the search for alternative causative mechanisms. Recently, a murine model of MAS induced by repeated stimulation of Toll-like receptor (TLR)-9 in genetically intact mice suggested that situations of continual activation of TLR-9 may reproduce the environment that leads to the development of MAS in the absence of known cytolytic defects.[39] Certain aspects of the disease in this model were interferon gamma (IFN-γ) dependent, establishing a connection to FHLH.[39]

The key role of IFN-γ in HLH was previously highlighted by the observation that, in perforin-deficient mice, only the antibody directed to IFN-γ, and not to other cytokines tested, prolonged survival and prevented the development of histiocytic infiltrates and cytopenia.[40] Furthermore, a study of liver biopsies in patients with various forms of HLH, including MAS, revealed extensive parenchymal infiltration by IFN-γ–producing CD8 T lymphocytes and hemophagocytic macrophages secreting tumor necrosis factor (TNF) alpha and interleukin (IL)-6.[41] Evidence has been provided that the hyperproduction of IL-18 (which potently induces Th-1 responses and IFN-γ production and enhances NK cell cytotoxicity) and an imbalance between levels of biologically active free IL-18 and those of its natural inhibitor (the IL-18 binding protein), may be involved in secondary hemophagocytic syndromes, including MAS.[42,43]

Another intriguing observation underscores the crucial regulatory role of IL-10 in the MAS process. Mice exposed to repeated TLR-9 stimulation coupled with blockade of the IL-10 receptor developed much more fulminant disease, including hemophagocytosis. This finding has led to the hypothesis that the combined immunologic abnormality of hyperactive TLR/IL-1β signaling and decreased IL-10 function may be responsible for a predisposition to MAS.[20] Altogether, the results of these studies highlight a critical importance of IFN-γ and IL-10 in the pathophysiology of HLH/MAS and provide the rationale for the modulation of the axes of these cytokines to treat disease.

CLINICAL, LABORATORY, AND HISTOPATHOLOGIC FEATURES

The clinical presentation of MAS is generally acute and may occasionally be dramatic, with the rapid development of multiorgan failure that requires the admission of the patient to the intensive care unit (ICU).[1,2] Fever is the main clinical manifestation of MAS. A useful clue to suspect the occurrence of MAS or to discriminate it from a flare of the underlying disease in a child with sJIA may be provided by the shift of fever from the high-spiking intermittent typical quotidian pattern of active sJIA to a continuous unremitting pattern characteristic of MAS. Other common clinical findings are hepatosplenomegaly and generalized lymphadenopathy, which are often present in active sJIA, but may worsen acutely at onset of MAS. Central nervous system (CNS) dysfunction is seen in approximately one-third of MAS cases and may cause lethargy, irritability, disorientation, headache, seizures, or coma. Importantly, CNS symptoms may uncover a coexistent thrombotic thrombocytopenic purpura. Approximately 20% of patients with MAS experience hemorrhagic manifestations, which may vary from easy bruising to purpura to mucosal bleeding. Heart, lung, and kidney failure is usually seen in the sickest patients, who are more likely to require admission to the ICU or have a fatal outcome. Recently, multiorgan failure, together with CNS involvement, hemoglobin level less than or equal to 7.9 g/dL, and age at onset of MAS greater than 11.5 years, was found to be an independent predictor of severity of the clinical course of MAS.[17] A few patients have pulmonary arterial hypertension, which is a serious, and often fatal, complication of sJIA that has frequently been observed in association with MAS.[44]

Typical laboratory abnormalities of MAS include a profound decrease in all 3 blood cell lines, with leukopenia, anemia, and thrombocytopenia. Liver function tests disclose frequently high levels of serum transaminases and, occasionally, increased bilirubin level. Moderate hypoalbuminemia is common. There is often an abnormal coagulation profile, with prolongation of prothrombin and partial thromboplastin times, hypofibrinogenemia, detectable fibrin degradation products, and increase in D-dimers. Additional laboratory findings include increased levels of triglycerides, lactate dehydrogenase, and ferritin. Serum ferritin is a valuable diagnostic tool, because the onset of MAS is often marked by a sharp increase of this biomarker, often to more than 5000 to 10,000 ng/mL. Measurement of the ferritin level over time may also assist in monitoring the course of disease activity, in assessing therapeutic response, and in predicting prognosis.[45] It has recently been proposed that the measurement of the soluble IL-2 receptor alpha chain (also known as soluble CD25) and soluble CD163, which may reflect the degree of activation and expansion of T cells and macrophages, respectively, are promising diagnostic markers for MAS and may help to identify subclinical forms.[15] However, these tests are not routinely performed or available in most pediatric rheumatology centers.

Another useful diagnostic hint is that patients may show a paradoxic improvement in the underlying inflammatory disease at the onset of MAS, with disappearance of signs and symptoms of arthritis and a decrease in the erythrocyte sedimentation rate (ESR). The latter phenomenon is mainly related to the hypofibrinogenemia secondary to fibrinogen consumption and liver dysfunction.[1] The ferritin/ESR ratio is a valuable tool in assessing MAS in sJIA.[46] Although the ESR decreases, the C-reactive protein level continues to increase with worsening MAS, and it has been shown that complement levels also decrease in patients with sJIA with active MAS.[47]

It is widely recognized that early suspicion of MAS is most commonly raised by the detection of subtle laboratory alterations, whereas clinical symptoms are often delayed.[46] However, the change in laboratory values over time is known to be more relevant for making an early diagnosis than their decrease below or increase above a certain threshold, as defined by current diagnostic guidelines[48,49] (discussed later). The performance of laboratory markers in the detection of MAS has been scrutinized recently by evaluating the change in value that takes place during the course of the syndrome. The tests that showed a percentage change greater than 50% between pre-MAS visit and MAS onset were the following: platelet count, aspartate and alanine aminotransferases, ferritin, lactate dehydrogenase, triglycerides, and D-dimer.[16]

A characteristic feature of MAS may be seen on bone marrow examination, which reveals numerous morphologically benign macrophages showing hemophagocytic activity. Such cells may infiltrate the lymph nodes and spleen as well as many other organs in the body and may be responsible for several clinical manifestations of the syndrome. However, in patients with MAS, the bone marrow aspirate does not always show hemophagocytosis (present in approximately 60% of patients).[16] Therefore, failure to reveal hemophagocytosis does not exclude the diagnosis of MAS.

Box 1 shows the main clinical and laboratory features of MAS complicating sJIA. The comparison of the features of active sJIA and MAS is presented in **Table 1**.

TRIGGERING FACTORS

Although most instances of MAS lack an identifiable precipitating factor, the syndrome has been associated with several triggers, including a flare of the underlying disease; toxicity of aspirin or other nonsteroidal antiinflammatory drugs; viral, bacterial, or fungal infections; a second injection of gold salts; or a side effect of second-line or biologic medications.[45,50,51] Severe episodes of MAS have been observed among patients who had undergone autologous bone marrow transplantation for sJIA refractory to conventional therapies.[52]

In the aforementioned multinational patient series,[16] MAS was reported to occur most frequently (51.7%) in the setting of active sJIA or during an sJIA flare. In 22.2% of the patients, MAS was diagnosed simultaneously with sJIA. An infectious trigger was detected in 34.1% of patients. Epstein-Barr virus (EBV) was the most

Box 1
Main features of MAS
Clinical features
Nonremitting fever
Hepatomegaly
Splenomegaly
Lymphadenopathy
Hemorrhagic manifestations
Encephalopathy
Laboratory features
Cytopenias
Abnormal liver function tests
Coagulopathy
Decreased ESR
Hypertriglyceridemia
Increased lactate dehydrogenase level
Hyponatremia
Hypoalbuminemia
Hyperferritinemia
Increased soluble IL-2 receptor alpha (or soluble CD25)
Increased soluble CD163
Histopathologic features
Macrophage hemophagocytosis in the bone marrow
Increased CD163 staining of bone marrow

Table 1
Comparison of clinical and laboratory features of active sJIA and MAS

Feature	sJIA	MAS
Fever pattern	Intermittent	Continuous
Rash	Maculopapular, evanescent	Petechial or purpuric
Hepatosplenomegaly	+	++
Lymphoadenopathy	+	++
Splenomegaly	+	++
Arthritis	++	−
Serositis	+	−
Hemorrhages	−	+
Encephalopathy	−	+
White blood cells and neutrophils	↑↑	↓
Hemoglobin	Normal or ↓	↓
Platelets	↑↑	↓
ESR	↑↑	Normal or ↓
Liver transaminases	Normal	↑↑
Bilirubin	Normal	Normal or ↑
Lactate dehydrogenase	Normal or ↑	↑↑
Triglycerides	Normal	↑
Prothrombin time	Normal	↑
Partial thromboplastin time	Normal	↑
Fibrinogen	↑	↓
D-dimer	↑	↑↑
Ferritin	Normal or ↑	↑↑
Soluble IL-2 receptor alpha (or soluble CD25)	Normal or ↑	↑↑
Soluble CD163	Normal or ↑	↑↑

common causative agent (25% of cases) among the 24 patients in whom the specific cause or the type of infection was identified or reported. In 3.8% of cases MAS was thought to be related to a medication side effect: 8 of the 11 instances involved a biologic agent, which was an IL-1 or IL-6 inhibitor in all but 1 case.

Induction of MAS by biologic agents that inhibit proinflammatory cytokines known to be involved in its pathogenesis is a paradoxic phenomenon. Suggested explanations include the increased rate of infections (which, in turn, may trigger MAS) associated with biologic therapies or the induction of an unbalance between upregulation and downregulation of the various molecules that are part of the cytokine network.[16,53] However, the proinflammatory cytokines might also be overwhelming the therapy because increasing IL-1 blockade has resolved MAS in children with sJIA who developed MAS while on IL-1 inhibitory therapy.[54]

DIAGNOSTIC GUIDELINES

MAS is a serious condition that, if untreated, may result in progressive multiorgan failure and eventual death. A mortality of 8% was recently reported.[16] A timely diagnosis and prompt initiation of appropriate treatment are, therefore, fundamental. However, early recognition of MAS is often challenging because there is no single pathognomonic clinical or laboratory parameter to aid in diagnosis. Furthermore, hemophagocytosis may not be seen in the initial stages[55] and lacks specificity for hemophagocytic syndromes.[56] In addition, the features of MAS may be hard to distinguish from those of conditions that may present with overlapping manifestations, such as flares of sJIA or systemic infections. The diagnostic difficulties are compounded by the variability in the potential severity of the syndrome and the heterogeneity of its clinical spectrum.[17]

The difficulties in making the diagnosis emphasize the importance of reliable criteria that aid physicians in identifying MAS in its earliest stages and distinguishing it from other conditions. The recognition that the syndrome is clinically similar to HLH has led some clinicians to recommend the use of the often restrictive HLH-2004 criteria.[21] An alternative approach is based on the application of the preliminary diagnostic guidelines for MAS complicating sJIA (**Box 2**).

Although both guidelines are considered potentially suitable for detecting MAS in sJIA, it has been argued that each of them is affected by several potential shortcomings.[20,49,57] The main limitation of using the HLH-2004 guidelines is thought to be that some individual criteria may not apply to patients with sJIA. Owing to the prominent inflammatory nature of sJIA, the occurrence of a relative reduction in white blood cell count, platelet level, or fibrinogen level rather that the absolute decrease required by the HLH-2004 criteria may be more useful to make an early diagnosis. In addition, the minimum threshold level for hyperferritinemia required for the diagnosis of HLH (500 ng/mL) may not be suitable to detect MAS in children with sJIA. It is well known that many patients with active sJIA, in the absence of MAS, have ferritin levels above that threshold.[58] In the acute phase of MAS, ferritin levels may peak at greater than 5000 ng/mL. Thus, a 500-ng/mL threshold may not discriminate MAS from a flare of

---

Box 2
Preliminary diagnostic guidelines for MAS complicating sJIA

Laboratory criteria

1. Decreased platelet count ($\leq$262 × 10^9/L)

2. Increased levels of aspartate aminotransferase (>59 U/L)

3. Decreased white blood cell count ($\leq$4.0 × 10^9/L)

4. Hypofibrinogenemia ($\leq$2.5 g/L)

Clinical criteria

1. CNS dysfunction (irritability, disorientation, lethargy, headache, seizures, coma)

2. Hemorrhages (purpura, easy bruising, mucosal bleeding)

3. Hepatomegaly ($\geq$3 cm below the costal arch)

Histopathologic criterion

Evidence of macrophage hemophagocytosis in the bone marrow aspirate

Diagnostic rule:

The diagnosis of MAS requires the presence of at least 2 laboratory criteria or the presence of at least 1 laboratory criterion and 1 clinical criterion. A bone marrow aspirate for the demonstration of hemophagocytosis may be required only in doubtful cases.

Adapted from Ravelli A, Magni-Manzoni S, Pistorio A, et al. Preliminary diagnostic guidelines for macrophage activation syndrome complicating systemic juvenile idiopathic arthritis. J Pediatr 2005;146(5):598–604.

sJIA. Other HLH criteria that are not readily applicable to MAS are the identification of low or absent NK cell activity or soluble cluster of differentiation 25 (sCD25) levels greater than the normal limits for age, because of the limited availability and lack of timeliness of these assays. The preliminary MAS guidelines have the disadvantage that the study that led to their development had insufficient data available for some important laboratory parameters of MAS; namely ferritin, triglycerides, and lactate dehydrogenase.

In a recent comparative analysis, the preliminary MAS guidelines performed better than the HLH-2004 guidelines in identifying MAS in the setting of sJIA, whereas the adapted HLH-2004 guidelines (with the exclusion of assessment of bone marrow hemophagocytosis, NK cell activity, and sCD25 levels) and the preliminary MAS guidelines with the addition of ferritin level greater than 500 ng/mL discriminated best between MAS and systemic infection.[59]

THE NEW CLASSIFICATION CRITERIA

An international collaborative effort to develop a set of classification criteria for MAS complicating sJIA has recently been reported. The criteria are based on a combination of expert consensus, available evidence from the medical literature, and analysis of real patient data (Ravelli A, Minoia F, Davì S, et al. Development and initial validation of classification criteria for macrophage activation syndrome complicating systemic juvenile idiopathic arthritis. Submitted for publication).[57] This project was conducted through the following steps: (1) Delphi survey among international pediatric rheumatologists designed to identify MAS features potentially suitable for inclusion in classification criteria, (2) large-scale data collection of patients with sJIA-associated MAS and 2 potentially confounding conditions, (3) Web-based consensus procedures among experts, (4) selection of candidate criteria through statistical analyses, and (5) selection of final classification criteria in a consensus conference.

The first step of the project was to identify candidate items using international consensus formation through the Delphi survey technique, and involved 232 pediatric rheumatologists from 47 countries. It led to the identification of 9 features that were thought by most of the respondents to be important as potential diagnostic criteria for MAS: declining platelet count, hyperferritinemia, evidence of macrophage hemophagocytosis in the bone marrow, increased serum liver enzyme levels, declining leukocyte count, persistent continuous fever greater than or equal to 38°C, decreasing ESR, hypofibrinogenemia, and hypertriglyceridemia.[60]

In the second phase, international pediatric rheumatologists and pediatric hematologist-oncologists were contacted by e-mail and invited to participate in a retrospective cohort study of patients with sJIA-associated MAS and with 2 conditions that could potentially be confused with MAS, represented by active sJIA not complicated by MAS and systemic infection.[16,17,59] The data for 1111 patients, 362 with sJIA-associated MAS, 404 with active sJIA without MAS, and 345 with systemic infection, were entered in the study Web site by 95 pediatric subspecialists practicing in 33 countries in 5 continents.

The final part of the project involved a panel of experts, composed of 20 pediatric rheumatologists and 8 pediatric hematologist-oncologists, selected because of their publication records and experience in the care of children with MAS and related disorders. The experts were first asked, through a series of Web-based consensus procedures, to classify a total of 428 patient profiles as having or not having MAS, based on the clinical and laboratory features recorded at disease onset. The profiles were selected randomly among the 1111 patients collected in the previous phase and comprised 161 patients with MAS, 140 patients with active sJIA without evidence of MAS, and 127 patients with systemic infection. The experts were purposely kept unaware of the original diagnosis as well as of the overall course of each patient. The minimum level of agreement among experts was set at 80%.

The best performing classification criteria were then selected by means of univariate and multivariate statistical analyses based on their ability to classify individual patients as having or not having MAS, using experts' diagnosis as the gold standard. Candidate classification criteria were partly derived from the literature and partly generated from the study data, by means of the combination of criteria approach or through multivariable logistic regression analyses, as reported (Ravelli A, Minoia F, Davì S, et al. Development and initial validation of classification criteria for macrophage activation syndrome complicating systemic juvenile idiopathic arthritis. Submitted for publication). A total of 982 candidate classification criteria were tested. For each set of criteria, the sensitivity, specificity, area under the receiver operating characteristic curve (AUC-ROC), and kappa value for agreement between the classification yielded by the criteria and the diagnosis of the experts were calculated. It was established that, in order to qualify for inclusion in expert voting procedures at the consensus conference, a set of classification criteria should show a kappa value greater than or equal to 0.85, a sensitivity greater than or equal to 0.80, a specificity greater than or equal to 0.93, and an AUC-ROC greater than or equal to 0.90. An exception was made for the historical literature criteria, which were retained for further consideration even if they did not meet all statistical requirements. Forty-five criteria were retained for further evaluation in the consensus conference.

The International Consensus Conference on MAS Classification Criteria was held in Genoa, Italy, on March 21 to 22, 2014, and was attended by all 28 experts who participated in Web-consensus evaluations. Attendees were randomized into 2 equally sized nominal groups and, using the nominal group technique, were asked to decide, independently of each other, which of the classification criteria that met the statistical requirements discussed earlier were easiest to use and most credible (ie, had the best face/content validity). A series of repeated independent voting sessions were held until the top 3 classification criteria were selected by each voting group. Then, an 80% consensus was attained on the best (final) set of classification criteria in a session with the 2 tables combined (**Box 3**).

MANAGEMENT

Because no controlled studies on the treatment of MAS are available, the management of this condition is largely empiric and based on anecdotal experience. The mainstay of

---

Box 3
The classification criteria for MAS in sJIA

A febrile patient with known or suspected sJIA is classified as having MAS if the following criteria are met:

Ferritin level greater than 684 ng/mL and any 2 of the following:

Platelet count less than or equal to 181×10^9/L

Aspartate aminotransferase level greater than 48 U/L

Triglyceride level greater than 156 mg/dL

Fibrinogen level less than or equal to 360 mg/dL

the therapy is traditionally constituted by the parenteral administration of high doses of corticosteroids. However, some fatalities have been reported among patients treated with massive doses of corticosteroids.[1,2] In the mid 1990s, the use of cyclosporine was advocated owing to its demonstrated benefit in the management of FHLH.[10] The observation of the marked efficacy of cyclosporine in some cases of MAS refractory to corticosteroids[61,62] has led to its proposed use as first-line treatment in MAS.[1,42] The experience with high-dose intravenous immunoglobulin, cyclophosphamide, plasma exchange, and etoposide has provided conflicting results. Etoposide is part of the protocol developed for treating FHLH.[21] However, it has been argued that, because this protocol carries a significant risk of mortality both before and after bone marrow transplantation, it may not be appropriate as first-line therapy for MAS as part of sJIA.[20] Whether or not a less aggressive use of etoposide for treating secondary forms of MAS, such as those complicating sJIA, will be beneficial remains unclear.

With the recent introduction of a variety of biologic agents, novel therapeutic approaches are being evaluated for MAS. The demonstration of increased production of TNF in the acute stage of MAS has provided the rationale for proposing inhibitors of this cytokine as potential therapeutic agents. However, although Prahalad and colleagues[63] reported the efficacy of etanercept in a boy with MAS, other investigators have observed the onset of MAS in patients with sJIA who were receiving etanercept.[64] The reports of MAS in the setting of TNF inhibition, together with the observations of a poorer efficacy of these biologic response modifiers in treating sJIA, has led to the assumption that this therapy may not be ideal for MAS occurring in children with sJIA.[20]

Recently, several cases have been reported of patients with sJIA-associated MAS who benefited dramatically from the administration of the IL-1 inhibitor, anakinra, after inadequate response to corticosteroids and cyclosporine.[65–68] However, there has been the suspicion that anakinra triggered MAS in 2 children with sJIA,[68,69] although the cause-effect relationship is difficult to establish. In a large case series of 46 patients with sJIA treated with anakinra at disease onset, this medication seemed to act as a potential MAS trigger in 5 children.[54] However, increased dosing of anakinra resolved MAS is most cases.[54] Thus, although the published experience has been favorable, more information is needed to define the role of IL-1 blockade therapy for the treatment of refractory MAS as part of sJIA.

Similar to IL-1 inhibition, IL-6 blockade through the anti–IL-6 receptor monoclonal antibody tocilizumab has proved highly efficacious in treating sJIA.[70] Whether tocilizumab will be similarly helpful in treating MAS is unclear at present, because there has been a case of MAS attributed to anti–IL-6 therapy.[71] Costimulatory blockade with cytotoxic T-lymphocyte-associated protein 4-Immunoglobulin (CTLA-4-Ig) has been beneficial anecdotally in children with severe sJIA with MAS,[72] but its place in treating MAS remains unknown.

A more aggressive intervention using antithymocyte globulin (ATG) has been used successfully in 2 patients with probable MAS.[73] However, ATG use carries a significant risk of serious infection and mortality.[74] The B cell–depleting anti-CD20 antibody rituximab has recently been reported to lead to remission in a sizable percentage of children with refractory sJIA.[75] Furthermore, this medication has anecdotally been used effectively to treat EBV-associated HLH/MAS in the setting of EBV infection.[76,77] However, to date no cases of rituximab therapy for MAS associated with sJIA have been reported.

In summary, there is increasing evidence that biologic therapies, particularly IL-1 inhibitors, represent a valuable adjunct to corticosteroids and cyclosporine in treating MAS associated with sJIA. Ongoing clinical experience and future pathogenetic studies will help to define the place of biologic therapies in management of MAS in children with sJIA.

REFERENCES

1. Ravelli A, Martini A. Macrophage activation syndrome. In: Lehman TH, Cimaz R, editors. Pediatric rheumatology. Amsterdam: Elsevier; 2008. p. 55–63.
2. Grom AA. Macrophage activation syndrome. In: Cassidy J, Petty RE, editors. Textbook of pediatric rheumatology. 6th edition. Philadelphia: Saunders Elsevier; 2010. p. 674–81.
3. Bae CB, Jung JY, Kim HA, et al. Reactive hemophagocytic syndrome in adult-onset Still disease: clinical features, predictive factors, and prognosis in 21 patients. Medicine (Baltimore) 2015;94(4):e451.
4. Parodi A, Davi S, Pringe AB, et al. Macrophage activation syndrome in juvenile systemic lupus erythematosus: a multinational multicenter study of thirty-eight patients. Arthritis Rheum 2009;60(11):3388–99.
5. Lambotte O, Khellaf M, Harmouche H, et al. Characteristic and long-term outcome of 15 episodes of systemic lupus erythematosus-associated hemophagocytic syndrome. Medicine (Baltimore) 2006;85(3):169–82.
6. Simonini G, Pagnini I, Innocenti L, et al. Macrophage activation syndrome/hemophagocytic lymphohistiocytosis and Kawasaki disease. Pediatr Blood Cancer 2010;55(3):592.
7. Rigante D, De Rosa G, Bertoni B, et al. Large pericardial effusion requiring pericardiocentesis as cardinal sign of macrophage activation syndrome in systemic onset-juvenile idiopathic arthritis. Rheumatol Int 2007;27(8):767–70.
8. Rossi-Semerano L, Hermeziu B, Fabre M, et al. Macrophage activation syndrome revealing familial Mediterranean fever. Arthritis Care Res (Hoboken) 2011;63(5): 780–3.
9. Hadchouel M, Prieur AM, Griscelli C. Acute hemorrhagic, hepatic and neurologic manifestations in juvenile rheumatoid arthritis: possible relationship to drugs or infection. J Pediatr 1985;106:562–6.
10. Stephan JL, Zeller J, Hubert P, et al. Macrophage activation syndrome and rheumatic disease in childhood: a report of four new cases. Clin Exp Rheumatol 1993; 11(4):451–6.
11. Ramanan AV, Schneider R. Macrophage activation syndrome–what's in a name! J Rheumatol 2003;30:2513–6.
12. Filipovich AH. Hemophagocytic lymphohistiocytosis (HLH) and related disorders. Hematology Am Soc Hematol Educ Program 2009;127–31.
13. Favara BE, Feller AC, Pauli M, et al. Contemporary classification of histiocytic disorders. The WHO Committee On Histiocytic/Reticulum Cell Proliferations. Reclassification Working Group of the Histiocyte Society. Med Pediatr Oncol 1997;29(3):157–66.
14. Behrens EM, Beukelman T, Paessler M, et al. Occult macrophage activation syndrome in patients with systemic juvenile idiopathic arthritis. J Rheumatol 2007;34(5):1133–8.
15. Bleesing J, Prada A, Siegel DM, et al. The diagnostic significance of soluble CD163 and soluble interleukin-2 receptor alpha-chain in macrophage activation syndrome and untreated new-onset systemic juvenile idiopathic arthritis. Arthritis Rheum 2007;56(3):965–71.
16. Minoia F, Davi S, Horne A, et al. Clinical features, treatment and outcome of macrophage activation syndrome complicating systemic juvenile idiopathic arthritis: A multinational, multicenter study of 362 patients. Arthritis Rheumatol 2014;66(11):3160–9.
17. Minoia F, Davì S, Horne A, et al. Dissecting the heterogeneity of macrophage activation syndrome complicating systemic juvenile idiopathic arthritis. J Rheumatol 2015;42(6):994–1001.

18. Schulert GS, Grom AA. Pathogenesis of macrophage activation syndrome and potential for cytokine-directed therapies. Annu Rev Med 2015;66:145–59.

19. Weaver LK, Behrens EM. Hyperinflammation, rather than hemophagocytosis, is the common link between macrophage activation syndrome and hemophagocytic lymphohistiocytosis. Curr Opin Rheumatol 2014;26(5):562–9.

20. Ravelli A, Grom AA, Behrens EM, et al. Macrophage activation syndrome as part of systemic juvenile idiopathic arthritis: diagnosis, genetics, pathophysiology and treatment. Genes Immun 2012;13(4):289–98.

21. Henter JI, Horne A, Arico M, et al. HLH-2004: diagnostic and therapeutic guidelines for hemophagocytic lymphohistiocytosis. Pediatr Blood Cancer 2007;48(2):124–31.

22. Sullivan KE, Delaat CA, Douglas SD, et al. Defective natural killer cell function in patients with hemophagocytic lymphohistiocytosis and in first degree relatives. Pediatr Res 1998;44(4):465–8.

23. Stepp SE, Dufourcq-Lagelouse R, Deist FL, et al. Perforin gene defects in familial hemophagocytic lymphohistiocytosis. Science 1999;286(5446):1957–9.

24. Feldmann J, Callebaut I, Raposo G, et al. Munc13-4 is essential for cytolytic granules fusion and is mutated in a form of familial hemophagocytic lymphohistiocytosis (FHL3). Cell 2003;115(4):461–73.

25. Zur SU, Rohr J, Seifert W, et al. Familial hemophagocytic lymphohistiocytosis type 5 (FHL-5) is caused by mutations in Munc18-2 and impaired binding to syntaxin 11. Am J Hum Genet 2009;85(4):482–92.

26. Zur SU, Schmidt S, Kasper B, et al. Linkage of familial hemophagocytic lymphohistiocytosis (FHL) type-4 to chromosome 6q24 and identification of mutations in syntaxin 11. Hum Mol Genet 2005;14(6):827–34.

27. Janka G, Zur SU. Familial and acquired hemophagocytic lymphohistiocytosis. Hematology Am Soc Hematol Educ Program 2005;82–8.

28. Jenkins MR, Rudd-Schmidt JA, Lopez JA, et al. Failed CTL/NK cell killing and cytokine hypersecretion are directly linked through prolonged synapse time. J Exp Med 2015;212(3):307–17.

29. Grom AA, Mellins ED. Macrophage activation syndrome: advances towards understanding pathogenesis. Curr Opin Rheumatol 2010;22(5):561–6.

30. Grom AA. Natural killer cell dysfunction: A common pathway in systemic-onset juvenile rheumatoid arthritis, macrophage activation syndrome, and hemophagocytic lymphohistiocytosis? Arthritis Rheum 2004;50(3):689–98.

31. Grom AA, Villanueva J, Lee S, et al. Natural killer cell dysfunction in patients with systemic-onset juvenile rheumatoid arthritis and macrophage activation syndrome. J Pediatr 2003;142(3):292–6.

32. Vastert SJ, van WR, D'Urbano LE, et al. Mutations in the perforin gene can be linked to macrophage activation syndrome in patients with systemic onset juvenile idiopathic arthritis. Rheumatology (Oxford) 2010;49(3):441–9.

33. Villanueva J, Lee S, Giannini EH, et al. Natural killer cell dysfunction is a distinguishing feature of systemic onset juvenile rheumatoid arthritis and macrophage activation syndrome. Arthritis Res Ther 2005;7(1):R30–7.

34. Hazen MM, Woodward AL, Hofmann I, et al. Mutations of the hemophagocytic lymphohistiocytosis-associated gene UNC13D in a patient with systemic juvenile idiopathic arthritis. Arthritis Rheum 2008;58(2):567–70.

35. Zhang M, Behrens EM, Atkinson TP, et al. Genetic defects in cytolysis in macrophage activation syndrome. Curr Rheumatol Rep 2014;16(9):439.

36. Spessott WA, Sanmillan ML, McCormick ME, et al. Hemophagocytic lymphohistiocytosis caused by dominant-negative mutations in STXBP2 that inhibit SNARE-mediated membrane fusion. Blood 2015;125(10):1566–77.

37. Yanagimachi M, Goto H, Miyamae T, et al. Association of IRF5 polymorphisms with susceptibility to hemophagocytic lymphohistiocytosis in children. J Clin Immunol 2011;31(6):946–51.

38. Kaufman KM, Linghu B, Szustakowski JD, et al. Whole-exome sequencing reveals overlap between macrophage activation syndrome in systemic juvenile idiopathic arthritis and familial hemophagocytic lymphohistiocytosis. Arthritis Rheumatol 2014;66(12):3486–95.

39. Behrens EM, Canna SW, Slade K, et al. Repeated TLR9 stimulation results in macrophage activation syndrome-like disease in mice. J Clin Invest 2011; 121(6):2264–77.

40. Jordan MB, Hildeman D, Kappler J, et al. An animal model of hemophagocytic lymphohistiocytosis (HLH): CD8+ T cells and interferon gamma are essential for the disorder. Blood 2004;104(3):735–43.

41. Billiau AD, Roskams T, Van Damme-Lombaerts R, et al. Macrophage activation syndrome: characteristic findings on liver biopsy illustrating the key role of activated, IFN-gamma-producing lymphocytes and IL-6- and TNF-a-producing macrophages. Blood 2005;105(4):1648–51.

42. Maeno N, Takei S, Nomura Y, et al. Highly elevated serum levels of interleukin-18 in systemic juvenile idiopathic arthritis but not in other juvenile idiopathic arthritis subtypes or in Kawasaki disease: comment on the article by Kawashima, et al. Arthritis Rheum 2002;46(9):2539–41.

43. Mazodier K, Marin V, Novick D, et al. Severe imbalance of IL-18/IL-18BP in patients with secondary hemophagocytic syndrome. Blood 2005;106(10): 3483–9.

44. Kimura Y, Weiss JE, Haroldson KL, et al. Pulmonary hypertension and other potentially fatal pulmonary complications in systemic juvenile idiopathic arthritis. Arthritis Care Res (Hoboken) 2013;65(5):745–52.

45. Ravelli A. Macrophage activation syndrome. Curr Opin Rheumatol 2002;14(5): 548–52.

46. Gorelik M, Fall N, Altaye M, et al. Follistatin-like protein 1 and the ferritin/erythrocyte sedimentation rate ratio are potential biomarkers for dysregulated gene expression and macrophage activation syndrome in systemic juvenile idiopathic arthritis. J Rheumatol 2013;40(7):1191–9.

47. Gorelik M, Torok KS, Kietz DA, et al. Hypocomplementemia associated with macrophage activation syndrome in systemic juvenile idiopathic arthritis and adult onset Still's disease: 3 cases. J Rheumatol 2011;38(2):396–7.

48. Lehmberg K, Pink I, Eulenburg C, et al. Differentiating macrophage activation syndrome in systemic juvenile idiopathic arthritis from other forms of hemophagocytic lymphohistiocytosis. J Pediatr 2013;162(6):1245–51.

49. Kelly A, Ramanan AV. Recognition and management of macrophage activation syndrome in juvenile arthritis. Curr Opin Rheumatol 2007;19(5):477–81.

50. Ruperto N, Brunner HI, Quartier P, et al. Two randomized trials of canakinumab in systemic juvenile idiopathic arthritis. N Engl J Med 2012;367(25):2396–406.

51. De Benedetti F, Brunner HI, Ruperto N, et al. Randomized trial of tocilizumab in systemic juvenile idiopathic arthritis. N Engl J Med 2012;367(25):2385–95.

52. De Kleer IM, Brinkman DM, Ferster A, et al. Autologous stem cell transplantation for refractory juvenile idiopathic arthritis: analysis of clinical effects, mortality, and transplant related morbidity. Ann Rheum Dis 2004;63(10):1318–26.

53. Buoncompagni A, Loy A, Sala I, et al. The paradox of macrophage activation syndrome triggered by biologic medications. Pediatr Rheumatol Online J 2005;3: 70–3.

54. Nigrovic PA, Mannion M, Prince FH, et al. Anakinra as first-line disease-modifying therapy in systemic juvenile idiopathic arthritis: report of forty-six patients from an international multicenter series. Arthritis Rheum 2011;63(2):545–55.
55. Arico M, Janka G, Fischer A, et al. Hemophagocytic lymphohistiocytosis. Report of 122 children from the International Registry. FHL Study Group of the Histiocyte Society. Leukemia 1996;10(2):197–203.
56. Ho C, Yao X, Tian L, et al. Marrow assessment for hemophagocytic lymphohistiocytosis demonstrates poor correlation with disease probability. Am J Clin Pathol 2014;141:62–71.
57. Davì S, Lattanzi B, Demirkaya E, et al. Toward the development of new diagnostic criteria for macrophage activation syndrome in systemic juvenile idiopathic arthritis. Ann Paediatr Rheumatol 2012;1:1–7.
58. Pelkonen P, Swanljung K, Siimes MA. Ferritinemia as an indicator of systemic disease activity in children with systemic juvenile rheumatoid arthritis. Acta Paediatr Scand 1986;75(1):64–8.
59. Davi S, Minoia F, Pistorio A, et al. Performance of current guidelines for diagnosis of macrophage activation syndrome complicating systemic juvenile idiopathic arthritis. Arthritis Rheumatol 2014;66(10):2871–80.
60. Davi S, Consolaro A, Guseinova D, et al. An international consensus survey of diagnostic criteria for macrophage activation syndrome in systemic juvenile idiopathic arthritis. J Rheumatol 2011;38(4):764–8.
61. Mouy R, Stephan JL, Pillet P, et al. Efficacy of cyclosporine A in the treatment of macrophage activation syndrome in juvenile arthritis: report of five cases. J Pediatr 1996;129(5):750–4.
62. Ravelli A, De Benedetti F, Viola S, et al. Macrophage activation syndrome in systemic juvenile rheumatoid arthritis successfully treated with cyclosporine. J Pediatr 1996;128(2):275–8.
63. Prahalad S, Bove KE, Dickens D, et al. Etanercept in the treatment of macrophage activation syndrome. J Rheumatol 2001;28(9):2120–4.
64. Ramanan AV, Schneider R. Macrophage activation syndrome following initiation of etanercept in a child with systemic onset juvenile rheumatoid arthritis. J Rheumatol 2003;30(2):401–3.
65. Miettunen PM, Narendran A, Jayanthan A, et al. Successful treatment of severe paediatric rheumatic disease-associated macrophage activation syndrome with interleukin-1 inhibition following conventional immunosuppressive therapy: case series with 12 patients. Rheumatology (Oxford) 2011;50(2):417–9.
66. Bruck N, Suttorp M, Kabus M, et al. Rapid and sustained remission of systemic juvenile idiopathic arthritis-associated macrophage activation syndrome through treatment with anakinra and corticosteroids. J Clin Rheumatol 2011;17(1):23–7.
67. Kelly A, Ramanan AV. A case of macrophage activation syndrome successfully treated with anakinra. Nat Clin Pract Rheumatol 2008;4(11):615–20.
68. Lurati A, Teruzzi B, Salmaso A, et al. Macrophage activation syndrome (MAS) during anti-IL1 therapy (anakinra) in a patient affected by systemic juvenile arthritis (soJIA): a report and review of the literature. Pediatr Rheumatol Online J 2005;3:79–85.
69. Zeft A, Hollister R, LaFleur B, et al. Anakinra for systemic juvenile arthritis: the Rocky Mountain experience. J Clin Rheumatol 2009;15(4):161–4.
70. Yokota S, Imagawa T, Mori M, et al. Efficacy and safety of tocilizumab in patients with systemic-onset juvenile idiopathic arthritis: a randomised, double-blind, placebo-controlled, withdrawal phase III trial. Lancet 2008;371(9617):998–1006.

71. Kobayashi M, Takahashi Y, Yamashita H, et al. Benefit and a possible risk of to-cilizumab therapy for adult-onset Still's disease accompanied by macrophage-activation syndrome. Mod Rheumatol 2011;21(1):92–6.
72. Record JL, Beukelman T, Cron RQ. Combination therapy of abatacept and ana-kinra in children with refractory systemic juvenile idiopathic arthritis: a retrospective case series. J Rheumatol 2011;38(1):180–1.
73. Coca A, Bundy KW, Marston B, et al. Macrophage activation syndrome: serological markers and treatment with anti-thymocyte globulin. Clin Immunol 2009; 132(1):10–8.
74. Mahlaoui N, Ouachee-Chardin M, de Saint BG, et al. Immunotherapy of familial hemophagocytic lymphohistiocytosis with antithymocyte globulins: a single-center retrospective report of 38 patients. Pediatrics 2007;120(3):e622–8.
75. Alexeeva EI, Valieva SI, Bzarova TM, et al. Efficacy and safety of repeat courses of rituximab treatment in patients with severe refractory juvenile idiopathic arthritis. Clin Rheumatol 2011;30(9):1163–72.
76. Balamuth NJ, Nichols KE, Paessler M, et al. Use of rituximab in conjunction with immunosuppressive chemotherapy as a novel therapy for Epstein Barr virus-associated hemophagocytic lymphohistiocytosis. J Pediatr Hematol Oncol 2007;29(8):569–73.
77. Bosman G, Langemeijer SM, Hebeda KM, et al. The role of rituximab in a case of EBV-related lymphoproliferative disease presenting with haemophagocytosis. Neth J Med 2009;67(8):364–5.

The Role of Hematopoietic Stem Cell Transplantation in Treatment of Hemophagocytic Lymphohistiocytosis

CrossMark

Sarah Nikiforow, MD, PhD

KEYWORDS

- Hemophagocytic lymphohistiocytosis • Stem cell transplantation • Alemtuzumab
- Chimerism • Treatment

KEY POINTS

- In cases of familial or relapsed/refractory HLH, hematopoietic stem cell transplant (HSCT) is indicated for optimal survival.
- Seventy-one percent of patients with pediatric/familial HLH for whom transplant is indicated are able to undergo HSCT. Long-term survival of children who undergo transplant is 66%.
- Use of alemtuzumab before conditioning favorably impacts donor chimerism and is becoming standard peritransplant therapy.
- Adult-onset HLH is increasingly recognized, and patients often bear classical familial HLH-associated genetic variants.
- The role of HSCT in adults, particularly older adults, is unclear, but overall outcomes after HSCT are encouraging.

INTRODUCTION

Hemophagocytic lymphohistiocytosis (HLH) was initially described as an inflammatory condition affecting young children with an abysmal prognosis. Early introduction of chemotherapeutic and immunomodulatory agents to suppress the unbridled yet ineffective phagocytic, natural killer (NK), and T-cell activity of HLH through the HLH-94 protocol had a dramatic impact on survival. To consolidate disease remission, children with familial, genetically based HLH and those with relapsed or primary refractory HLH require allogeneic hematopoietic stem cell transplantation (HSCT).

Stem Cell Transplantation Program, Cell Manipulation Core Facility, Dana-Farber Cancer Institute, Dana 168, 450 Brookline Avenue, Boston, MA 02215, USA
E-mail address: Sarah_Nikiforow@DFCI.HARVARD.EDU

Hematol Oncol Clin N Am 29 (2015) 943–959
http://dx.doi.org/10.1016/j.hoc.2015.06.011
0889-8588/15/$ – see front matter © 2015 Elsevier Inc. All rights reserved.

Introduction of alemtuzumab into the peritransplant regimen is under investigation to improve chimerism and other clinical outcomes. Unfortunately, the role of stem cell transplantation in adults with HLH is not as clear-cut. HLH often presents in adults in concert with an underlying malignancy and may shift the decision to pursue alloge- neic HSCT sooner in the cancer treatment algorithm. When adults present with HLH without an accompanying lymphoma or leukemia, decisions to pursue HSCT are individualized and, unfortunately, not informed by adequate published data. At our institution, this decision is made based on the constellation of underlying muta- tions/genetic variants, aspects of the HLH remission after therapy, and donor availability.

ACHIEVING REMISSION IN PEDIATRIC HEMOPHAGOCYTIC LYMPHOHISTIOCYTOSIS

Familial HLH was initially described by Farquhar and Claireaux[1] in two infant sib- lings who both had a rapidly fatal clinical course. Over the succeeding decades, ge- netic underpinnings of the disease in familial cases were described, namely autosomal-recessive mutations at 9q21.3-locus 6 and in perforin, MUNC 13–4, Syn- taxin 11, and Syntaxin Binding Protein 2/MUNC 18 to two genes. These mutations affect cytotoxic granule composition, transport, and release. They result in impaired apoptosis and a vicious cytokine-driven, cell-mediated inflammatory response.[2] Provoking infectious agents, particularly those of the herpes virus family, were iden- tified. Lymphocyte-directed chemotherapy and immunotherapy were noted to have some efficacy in small studies, but children with familial HLH all experienced relapse.

The Histiocyte Society's prospective international therapeutic study, HLH-94, rep- resented the first large effort to systematically define the disease and implement a standardized therapeutic strategy.[3] On this study, children younger than 15 years of age were treated with 8 weeks of induction therapy consisting of tapering dexameth- asone doses, etoposide, and intrathecal methotrexate. Patients with no evidence of familial disease who showed disease resolution after the 8-week induction period were followed but did not continue to further therapy unless reactivation occurred. For patients with familial, clinically persistent, or relapsing disease, continuation ther- apy consisting of dexamethasone pulses, etoposide doses every 2 weeks, and cyclo- sporine was recommended. Allogeneic HSCT was pursued in those patients for whom a suitable donor was available.

Long-term results of this study, representing a cohort of 227 patients with greater than or equal to 5 years follow-up, demonstrated that 86% of patients were alive after the 8-week induction course; 59% of these had no signs of active disease.[4] Children who did not survive the induction period were more likely to have presented with hyperbilirubinemia, renal failure, and abnormal findings on brain imaging. Notable characteristics of patients in this study included a median age of 8 months; 76% were younger than 2 years of age. Neurologic symptoms were present in 33% before therapy, and 46% had a history of recent infection. Familial disease was documented in 24%. Poor prognoses were associated with neurologic symptoms and central ner- vous system (CNS) pleocytosis at presentation and age less than 6 months. In this and subsequent studies, thrombocytopenia, initial or persistent ferritin levels greater than 2000 ng/mL, degree of soluble interleukin-2 receptor (sIL-2R) elevation, and the rate of decline of ferritin had prognostic implications. A ferritin decrease of less than 50% im- parts an odds ratio for death of 17 when compared with a ferritin decrease of greater than 95% during therapy.[5] Therapeutic guidelines and diagnostic criteria were further updated in the HLH-2004 treatment protocol, with primary changes being initiation of cyclosporine at the start of induction and specific guidelines on management of CNS disease.[6] An alternative induction regimen consisting of steroids, cyclosporine, and antithymocyte globulin (ATG) instead of etoposide has been investigated. A higher initial complete response rate of 73% was seen but so was a 25% rate of early relapse and death before subsequent therapies.[7,8]

For patients with either primary refractory or relapsing disease, multiple salvage therapies have been investigated. The best quantity and quality of data supports use of alemtuzumab, an antibody capable of rapidly and efficiently eliminating CD52-expressing cells, which include most mononuclear subsets (B-cell, T-cell, and NK cell lymphocytes, monocytes, macrophages, monocyte-derived dendritic cells, and eosinophils) but not hematopoietic stem cells.[9] Building on case reports, a retrospective analysis of 22 children and adults with refractory HLH manifested by elevated ferritin and sIL-2R levels, cytopenias, organomegaly, and/or continued hemophagocytosis was conducted. Alemtuzumab was introduced in dose-escalated, fixed dose, or individualized schema, either intravenously or subcutaneously.[10,11] The median alemtuzumab dose was 1 mg/kg (range, 0.1–8.9) over a median of 4 days (range, 2–10). Half of patients received subsequent additional courses of alemtuzumab. After 2 weeks, most patients experienced decreases in inflammatory markers: 67% of patients evaluable for ferritin had a greater than or equal to 25% decrease and 78% of patients evaluable for sIL-2R had a 1.6- to 4-fold decrease. Seventy-six percent of patients with neutropenia (ANC <2000 cells/μL) had increases in absolute neutrophil count (ANC). Liver function tests improved in all affected individuals. Unfortunately, no patient experienced a complete response to alemtuzumab therapy. There was no correlation of response with identification of a genetically predisposing mutation. Most patients went on to receive further definitive therapy. Nine of the 22 patients experienced bacteremia or candidemia, a third had cytomegalovirus viremia, a quarter had Epstein-Barr virus (EBV) viremia, and a quarter had adenovirus in the serum in the first few months following alemtuzumab therapy. Seventy-seven percent of patients survived to undergo HSCT.

Evidence for using other anti-inflammatory agents to block cytokines, macrophages, and/or T cells is based on case reports. Therapies have been successful in secondary HLH and macrophage activation syndrome arising out of rheumatologic disease using infliximab (anti–tumor necrosis factor-α), anakinra (anti–IL-1 receptor), tocilizumab (anti–IL-6), and daclizumab (anti-CD25). Success in these cases was defined as response of symptoms, tolerating a steroid taper, or survival to definitive therapy.[12–15] Splenectomy has also been investigated.[16] Long-term outcomes after these therapies followed by subsequent HSCT have not been studied in a systematic fashion.

RATIONALE FOR ALLOGENEIC HEMATOPOIETIC STEM CELL TRANSPLANTATION IN PEDIATRIC HEMOPHAGOCYTIC LYMPHOHISTIOCYTOSIS

Although there have been case reports of HSCT for HLH since 1986, the first series examining its use was published in 1991 in nine children with "familial HLH" based on their age of presentation. They were treated initially with etoposide, steroids, and intrathecal methotrexate.[17,18] Of 22 patients enrolled, 16 survived induction therapy, and 15 entered complete remission (CR). Ten of the patients in CR received maintenance chemotherapy. Six patients (five in CR, one in partial remission [PR]) underwent upfront stem cell transplant. Five had an HLA-matched sibling donor; one had a single antigen-mismatched parent as donor. Three additional children who relapsed on chemotherapy subsequently underwent HSCT from a two- or three-antigen mismatched parental donor while in PR. Conditioning consisted of a myeloablative regimen of cyclophosphamide, busulfan, and etoposide/VP-16 (CBV). All patients received bone marrow–derived stem cells. Notable findings were that 8 of 10 patients on maintenance chemotherapy relapsed in a mean of 5.4 months (range, 2–8 months), including four in the CNS. The two patients surviving after chemotherapy alone had no documented family history of HLH. Of the five children who underwent HSCT from a matched related donor (MRD), four were alive without therapy at more than 1 to 6 years. The recipient who relapsed had received stem cells from a sister who subsequently developed HLH herself. Of the four patients transplanted from non-HLA identical donors, one did not engraft and the other three had active disease at the time of transplant. All died of HLH progression. Restoration of normal NK cell activity after HSCT was seen in those with prolonged survival. This study established two tenets in treatment of pediatric HLH: chemotherapy alone is not sufficient for long-term control of familial HLH; and HSCT from a sibling donor improves survival for familial HLH. Other questions raised and under investigation in current trials were (1) what is the role of unrelated and mismatched donors in HLH, (2) how important is donor chimerism in maintaining remission after HSCT, (3) how crucial is disease activity at time of HSCT, and (4) how might inherited risk factors for HLH in an asymptomatic sibling donor impact prognosis in the recipient.

Confirming these observations, 48 children, 33 of whom had proven familial HLH and 15 with relapsed or refractory HLH, underwent HSCT after induction therapy with HLH-94 etoposide-based therapy or steroids, cyclosporine $\pm$ ATG.[19] A total of 56% were in CR, 34% in PR, and 10% had active disease at the time of HSCT. Fourteen had matched sibling donors and received T-cell replete marrows. The others received T-cell depleted transplants, four from matched unrelated donors (MUD), one from a two-antigen mismatched donor, and 29 from related haploidentical donors. Conditioning entailed myeloablative CBV or cyclophosphamide, busulfan, and ATG. Event-free survival was 58.5% with median follow-up of more than 5 years. Donor compatibility in this study had no significant impact on survival, except when HLH was active at transplant, in which case MRD and MUD recipients had improved outcomes ($P = .03$). There was a trend to worsened survival with uncontrolled HLH at time of HSCT ($P = .053$).

Several additional observations arose from this trial. One was a high rate of both primary graft failure and secondary graft rejection affecting 25% of patients. Active HLH at time of HSCT, older age of the recipient, and perhaps having a haploidentical donor were associated with primary graft failure. Twelve of the 15 patients with graft failure underwent a second transplant. The second was that HLH recurrence was the primary cause of death in 50% of cases. In 28 long-term survivors, 50% had full donor chimerism and 50% had mixed chimerism (<95% donor). When donor chimerism was greater than 10% to 20%, stable CR of HLH was maintained.

In the largest study of HLH pediatric patients to date involving 249 patients enrolled on HLH-94, 14% died during the initial induction period, primarily from active disease.[3,4] Overall survival (OS) at 5 years was 54%. One hundred twenty-four patients underwent HSCT, primarily with myeloablative CBV conditioning $\pm$ ATG. Five-year survival after HSCT was 66%. There was a trend to improved 5-year survival in patients with CR at HSCT (72%) versus those with active HLH (58%; $P = .064$). A total of 53 patients survived without HSCT. These patients were older (median age, 24 months); female; and less likely to have hepatomegaly, splenomegaly, persisting hyperferritinemia, or neurologic complications. Fifty-seven percent of patients surviving without HSCT were from Japan, and 52% had an infectious trigger, primarily EBV. None of those with familial HLH survived without HSCT.

ADVANCES IN CONDITIONING INTENSITY

In early studies of HSCT for HLH, toxicities with a myeloablative conditioning (MAC) regimen, usually CBV ± ATG, were significant. Small series investigated substituting total body irradiation for etoposide.[20] Toxicities included significant rates of veno-occlusive disease (28%–38%) particularly in haploidentical transplants, after ATG, and in patients younger than 12 months.[19] Rates of significant infections, especially viral infections, were 60% to 72%. Rates of acute graft-versus-host disease (GvHD) ranged from 17% to 44%; rate of chronic GvHD was 9%. In HLH-94, 29 of the 42 deaths after HSCT occurred in the first 100 days, and transplant-related mortality (TRM) affected 23% of recipients.[3,4] In one study, 50% of children required intensive care unit admission after MAC HSCT.[21] Long-term survival ranged from 45% to 65%.[22–24]

These rates of complications were higher than expected or acceptable in pediatric transplants, so reduced-intensity conditioning (RIC) regimens were investigated to decrease TRM while still resetting the immune dysregulation of HLH. Cooper and colleagues[25] first described 12 children who underwent RIC (primarily fludarabine, melphalan ± busulphan) and established feasibility. All patients in this series engrafted. Survival at a median of 30 months was 75% with all patients in CR, despite one-third of survivors having mixed chimerism. Rates of TRM, acute GvHD, and chronic GvHD were 25%, 33%, and 25%, respectively. In a subsequent update on a total of 25 patients, survival rates were 84% at a median of 3 years after HSCT.[26] Similar results were seen among 40 patients with familial HLH at Cincinnati Children's Hospital, 14 with MAC (CB + ATG ± etoposide) and 26 with RIC consisting of fludarabine, melphalan, and alemtuzumab.[27] Approximately 60% in each group were in CR at time of HSCT with a substantial portion (35%) of RIC patients having undergone salvage therapy with alemtuzumab before HSCT. Most patients received bone marrow stem cells from unrelated fully matched or single antigen-mismatched donors. Two patients received umbilical cord stem cells. Estimated 3-year survival was 43% after MAC and 92% after RIC (P = .0001). All patients engrafted. Rates of bacterial infections were 14% in MAC and 15% in RIC; rates of EBV, cytomegalovirus, adenoviral, and other viral infections/viremia were 29%, 29%, 15%, and 29% in MAC and 15%, 27%, 38%, and 8% in RIC, respectively. Grades II and III acute GvHD rates were 14% in MAC and 8% in RIC, without any grade IV acute GvHD seen. Chronic GvHD was not seen after MAC; 12% of RIC patients experienced limited chronic GvHD. Although not all studies replicate these findings of improved survival after RIC versus MAC regimens for HLH, the previously mentioned data have made HSCT with RIC the standard approach to familial, refractory, and relapsed pediatric HLH.[27,28] Specific chemotherapy and immunosuppression agents, such as fludarabine, melphalan, treosulfan, ATG, and alemtuzumab, have all been used in conditioning with similar success.[29,30]

USE OF ALTERNATIVE DONOR SOURCES

Given the familial clustering of HLH in pediatric cases, unrelated, mismatched, haploidentical, and umbilical cord donors have always been the main stem cell sources for HSCT. (Development of disease in initially unaffected sibling donors can be seen.) In the HLH-94 study, among 124 HSCT recipients, 5-year survival rates were 74% for MRD, 76% for MUD, 61% for mismatched unrelated donors (MMUD), 43% for haploidentical donors, and 80% for the 10 umbilical cord recipients.[4] Survival between MRD and MUD recipients was not significantly different. In a separate analysis of 86 children receiving HLH-94 followed by MAC HSCT, adjusted odds ratio for mortality were 1.93

(confidence interval, 0.61–6.19) for MUD, 3.31 (confidence interval, 1.02–10.76) for haploidentical donors, and 3.01 (confidence interval, 0.91–9.97) for MMUD when compared with MRD.[23] These trends have been recapitulated in smaller series.[31] Haploidentical donor sources were often associated with increased risk of graft failure.[19]

Experience with umbilical cord blood (UCB) stem cells has recently grown. Ohga and colleagues[28] found survival greater than 65% after cord transplant in 28 patients, both those with familial and EBV-triggered HLH; those patients received primarily MAC. In that study, the risk of death for familial HLH patients was marginally higher for those receiving cord (P = .07) versus MUD stem cells. Rates of engraftment were 60% and similar between stem cell sources. A recent study of 13 familial HLH patients confirmed the feasibility of RIC UCB transplants for HLH. Ten patients showed initial engraftment, two more engrafted after the second cord transplant, two had late graft failure, and two relapsed with HLH.[32] Thus, although not as well studied, UCB transplant seems feasible with outcomes similar to transplants from other unrelated stem cell sources.

SPECIFIC ROLE OF ALEMTUZUMAB AND IMPORT OF POST–HEMATOPOIETIC STEM CELL TRANSPLANTATION CHIMERISM

Alemtuzumab has been used in many stages of HLH, as salvage therapy and in HSCT conditioning. Studies of alemtuzumab demonstrate clear efficacy in patients with refractory disease with a 64% response rate and 77% rate of survival to HSCT.[11] All but one patient undergoing HSCT survived to Day 100 with an overall probability of long-term survival of 64%. Thus, in patients surviving the salvage regimen, outcome after HSCT is similar to those undergoing upfront transplantation.

Alemtuzumab has been successfully incorporated into RIC in place of ATG. But there is higher prevalence of persistent donor chimerism. Among 26 patients receiving fludarabine, melphalan, and alemtuzumab pre-HSCT, all engrafted but 65% showed mixed chimerism. Ouachée-Chardin and coworkers[19] demonstrated that CR was sustained as long as donor chimerism remained greater than 10% to 20% and patients did not experience secondary graft rejection. Six of 21 survivors after HSCT in the study by Cooper and colleagues[26] had mixed chimerism. All retained their grafts and stayed in remission, including one who had donor cells only in the T-cell compartment. The pathophysiology of early HLH recurrence in situations of waning chimerism is unknown, but some have cited persistence of host macrophages, NK cells, and T cells in combination with high incidence of viral reactivation early after HSCT as factors enabling recurrent immune dysregulation.

Given the high incidence of mixed chimerism with alemtuzumab and resulting concern for increased relapse, several interventions are used. Donor lymphocyte infusion (DLI) may be pursued when chimerism rapidly declines or drops below 40% to 60% within the first 6 months after HSCT. Marsh and colleagues[33] administered DLI (one to three doses) and/or CD34$^+$ stem cell boost to 14 of 17 patients with mixed chimerism after RIC HSCT. Five patients developed grade II or III acute GvHD after DLI. One patient who dropped to 9% donor chimerism experienced HLH recurrence. The rate of mixed chimerism was decreased (29% vs 79%; P = .0225) when alemtuzumab was delivered at higher dose farther before or "distal" to transplant (Days -22 to -19) as opposed to lower dose "proximal" administration (Days -12/8 to -9/4). However, acute GvHD was increased with distal dosing. To follow up this observation, an intermediate schedule of alemtuzumab dosed Day -14 to Day -10 before HSCT to a total of 1 mg/kg was compared retrospectively with proximal and distal administration involving several dosing schedules along with fludarabine and melphalan conditioning.[34] The 71 patients were children and young adults up to age 26; 43% had documented genetic diagnoses and an additional 6% were single heterozygotes for classical mutations. Seventy-six percent of patients received fully matched stem cells, 24% had MRDs, and almost all received bone marrow. With the caveat that a variety of doses and schedules were used within the proximal and distal cohorts, the intermediate group demonstrated reduced rates of mixed chimerism (31%) compared with the proximal group (72%; $P<.01$) and distal group receiving greater than or equal to 2 mg/kg alemtuzumab (75%; $P = .04$). Regarding dynamics of chimerism, only 13% in the intermediate alemtuzumab group dropped below 20% as compared with 25% of patients in the proximal and distal high-dose groups. Interventions pursued when donor chimerism dropped to less than 95% were withdrawal of immune suppression, followed by one or more DLIs at rates of 14%, 53% ($P = .01$), and 38% ($P = .02$) in the intermediate, proximal, and high-dose distal groups, respectively. These interventions resulted in more than 75% of patients maintaining more than 50% donor chimerism at last follow-up; four patients required a second allogeneic HSCT. Rates of grades II to IV acute GvHD after initial transplant were low at 0%, 4%, and 13% in the intermediate, proximal, and distal groups, respectively, and 8% to 14% after withdrawal of immune suppression ± DLI. In multivariable analysis, there were no significant differences in survival (80%–91% at 1 year and 80%–82% at last follow-up) based on alemtuzumab dosing schedule.

ALGORITHM FOR HEMATOPOIETIC STEM CELL TRANSPLANTATION FAMILIAL VERSUS INFECTION-ASSOCIATED HEMOPHAGOCYTIC LYMPHOHISTIOCYTOSIS

Thus, over the past three decades, the quarter of pediatric cases having genetically based, familial HLH has been systematically controlled with initial antilymphocyte therapy consisting of etoposide, cyclosporine, and steroids ± methotrexate. These patients require continuation therapy to temporize until up-front allogeneic stem cell transplant is undergone (**Fig. 1**). Patients with clinically refractory disease or who relapse after induction therapy (about a third of the presenting population) also should undergo stem cell transplantation. Over two-thirds of patients for whom transplant is recommended survive initial induction or salvage regimens. Overall about half of children with HLH end up undergoing allogeneic HSCT. Survival rates after RIC HSCT are more than 75%. Up to 20% of children will be alive and well without transplant.

How to stratify children who respond clinically but have very high initial elevations and/or a slow decline of ferritin or sIL-2R, indicating high risk for recurrence is unclear. Similarly, the role of HSCT in patients not in CR after induction but who achieve CR on continuation therapy is undefined. In the HLH-94 protocol, 76% of patients who had long-term disease-free survival without HSCT achieved CR in 2 months, but another 18% achieved CR in the following 4 months. Salvage regimens, such as alemtuzumab, are efficacious, but only in two-thirds of individuals who often do not achieve CR. Although CR at time of transplant correlated with improved prognosis after HSCT, outcomes justify taking those with PRs and active disease immediately into HSCT until more effective therapies can be identified.

Current practice is to pursue RIC from matched related, unrelated, mismatched, haploidentical, or cord sources. Trends toward improved survival are seen in fully matched settings. Lack of engraftment and secondary graft rejection encountered after RIC, particularly after UCB or haploidentical HSCT, can be managed by a second transplant. Increased rates and magnitude of residual host chimerism are addressed with pre-emptive DLI or CD34 boosts and modification of alemtuzumab dosing peritransplant. Although intermediate dosing of alemtumuzab (ie, 1 mg/kg starting Day

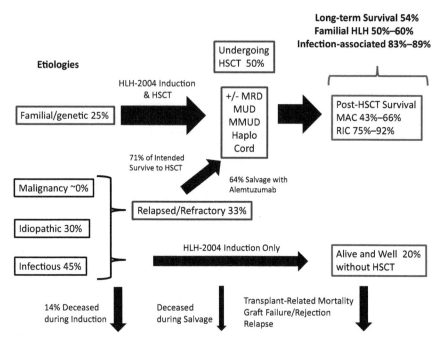

Fig. 1. Pediatric HLH treatment algorithm. Children presenting with familial or genetically driven HLH and those who manifest primary refractory or relapsed disease are recommended to undergo HSCT from fully matched or alternative stem cell sources, often with peri-transplant alemtuzumab. Children with idiopathic or infection-associated HLH are treated with standard etoposide, steroid, and calcineurin inhibitor therapy (HLH-94 or HLH-2004 regimens). Those who demonstrate a complete response are then observed. Approximate percentages of the pediatric HLH population presenting with each underlying cause and estimated survival on each therapeutic regimen are shown. Cord, umbilical cord unit; Haplo, haploidentical donor.

-14) has significantly reduced the incidence of, severity, and need for intervention in mixed chimerism, improvements in clinical end points, such as relapse or survival, have not been demonstrated. The multicenter phase II RICHI trial (CTN 1204, NCT 01998633 at clinicaltrials.gov) is currently enrolling children and young adults to age 35 with HLH or selected primary immunodeficiencies to a standardized RIC regimen of fludarabine, melphalan, and intermediate timing of alemtuzumab. If successful, this is likely to become a standard approach, at least within the United States.

Subgroups that deserve special mention are congenital immunodeficiencies, which entail high risk of HLH and EBV-associated HLH. For such diseases as X-linked lymphoproliferative disease (XLP1) caused by SAP/SH2D1A deficiency, Griscelli syndrome, and X-linked inhibitor of apoptosis protein deficiency (XIAP), presentation with HLH often portends a significantly worse prognosis. There is no consensus as to whether clinically stable patients with XLP1 should undergo HSCT. But mortality for patients presenting with HLH can be 66%, with survival of only 19% without allogeneic HSCT.[35] Survival of 50% with HSCT after HLH in one study and 71% in another confirms the role of transplant.[36] Similarly, patients with XIAP and HLH benefit from RIC HSCT, although survival is less than 50%. Here disease control was crucial to survival because no children entering HSCT with active HLH survived.[37]

Pediatric HLH triggered by infection, specifically by EBV, seems to be a significantly different entity, particularly in East and South Asian countries. In the HLH-94 experience, almost 60% of the patients well and off therapy without HSCT were from Japan and 50% had a clear infectious trigger to their HLH. In a separate study of 78 Japanese patients with EBV-associated HLH, only 18% proceeded to transplant; survival was 75% after HSCT.[38] Similarly, another Japanese study noted 83% and 89% 3-year survival for EBV and other infection-associated HLH versus 60% for familial HLH.[39] Therefore, most children with infection-associated HLH will not end up needing HSCT. One series of 23 cases of infection-associated HLH demonstrated excellent outcomes with steroids and supportive measures alone, highlighting the excellent prognosis and potentially reduced need for therapy for this subgroup.[40] In contrast, another study indicated that mortality rates were 14 times higher in children with EBV-associated HLH who were not given etoposide.[41]

UNIQUE ASPECTS OF ADULT-ONSET HEMOPHAGOCYTIC LYMPHOHISTIOCYTOSIS

"Acquired" or "secondary" HLH can be seen in all age groups but comprises most cases presenting in adulthood. Because HLH is more frequently recognized in adults, unique clinical, biochemical, immunologic, and genetic features that characterize adult presentation are becoming apparent. Adults now comprise up to 40% of HLH cases, with median age of diagnosis being mid-40s to 50s. Cases are even seen older than age 70. The incidence may be 1 in 2000 adult admissions at tertiary medical centers.[42] Although the HLH-94 and HLH-2004 diagnostic criteria were designed for children, nearly all adult patients reveal a similar constellation of features including fevers, cytopenias, phagocytosis, elevated ferritin, and sIL-2R. However, they manifest lower levels of splenomegaly, hypofibrinogenemia, hypertriglyceridemia, and poor correlation of disease with decreased or absent NK function.[43,44] Because acquired or reactive HLH in adults is clinically difficult to distinguish from severe sepsis or hematologic malignancy and has attributes distinct from pediatric presentations, metrics for diagnosis specific to adults have been sought. A novel scoring system called the HScore was recently developed and validated.[45] Three clinical variables (underlying immunosuppression, high temperature, and organomegaly) were combined with five biologic variables (triglyceride, ferritin, liver aspartate aminotransferase/alanine aminotransferase, fibrinogen, and cytopenias) and one cytologic variable (hemophagocytosis on bone marrow aspirate) and weighted. The probability of having HLH was less than 1% for an HScore of less than or equal to 90 and greater than 99% for an HScore of greater than or equal to 250. Levels of interferon-γ and IL-10 have also been investigated as diagnostic and prognostic tools for distinguishing HLH from sepsis and acute viral infections. Levels of interferon-γ greater than 75 pg/mL and IL-10 greater than 60 pg/mL have 99% sensitivity and 93% specificity for HLH, as compared with the isolated elevations of IL-6 seen in sepsis.[46] Patients with secondary HLH also have severe imbalances of IL-18 to IL-18 binding protein ratios, perhaps enabling Th1 lymphocyte and macrophage activation.

Other differences between pediatric and adult cases of HLH include lower sensitivity and specificity of ferritin levels greater than 10,000 ng/mL in adults. There is no documented prognostic import of rate of ferritin decline in adults. Malignancies, particularly B-cell and NK/T-cell lymphomas, underlie around 50% of cases of adult-onset HLH.[47] It is estimated that HLH affects 0.9% of all adults with hematologic malignancies and up to 20% of adults with certain B-cell lymphomas, NK/T-cell nasal lymphomas, and panniculitis-like T-cell lymphomas.[48] Several groups have identified biochemical features of adult HLH that correlate with underlying malignancy and thus indicate need for further diagnostic investigation. These include lower fibrinogen less than 1.5 g/L, lactate dehydrogenase greater than or equal to 1,000 U/L, an elevated sIL-2R/ferritin ratio, and in several studies platelets less than 40×10^9/L.[49]

To further complicate adult-onset HLH, homozygous, compound heterozygous, or single mutations/variations in classical FHLH genes are found in symptomatic and asymptomatic adults as genetic testing becomes more widely available. Children with mutations in the same gene can manifest different clinical presentations. FHLH-2 with canonical perforin mutations is typically characterized by early onset (<2 months of age), very high ferritin and sIL-2R levels, and persistent deficiencies in NK cell activity.[50] However, children with missense mutations in *PRF1* develop disease later and show only moderately reduced cytotoxicity. Patients with splice-site mutations in *STXBP2* versus nonsense mutations develop clinical manifestations at an older age (median, 4.1 years vs 2 months).[51] Recently, hypomorphic missense and splice-site variants in perforin (*PRF1*), syntaxin 11 (*STX11*), and syntaxin binding protein 2 (*STXBP2*) genes have been found in single heterozygous, compound heterozygous, and homozygous states in 14% of adults referred for genetic testing.[52]

The best studied of such single-nucleotide polymorphisms is the A91V *PRF1* variant. It is present in 4% to 7% of the general population yet has been correlated with absent or low levels of perforin expression and variability in cytotoxic function in some heterozygotes and homozygotes. Heterozygosity for the A91V variant is more frequent in patients with HLH and some lymphomas than in the normal population.[53–55] Of 24 A91V heterozygotes with HLH, 10 had additional mutations in either MUNC13 to 4 or perforin. Thus, A91V *PRF1* mutations may be permissive but not sufficient for development of HLH. How many of these individuals, particularly those with single variants, will eventually manifest clinical HLH or have a familial syndrome, and how many individuals harboring the same single-nucleotide polymorphism will never develop HLH is as yet unknown.

RATIONALE FOR ALLOGENEIC HEMATOPOIETIC STEM CELL TRANSPLANTATION IN ADULT HEMOPHAGOCYTIC LYMPHOHISTIOCYTOSIS

Most studies of adults show outcomes inferior to those in children, particularly for adults with malignancy-associated HLH. Among 1109 adult cases collated from numerous publications, the mortality rate was 41%.[47] In a Japanese study, 5-year OS was greater than 80% for patients with EBV- or other infection- and autoimmune-associated HLH, 48% to 54% for familial HLH or B-cell lymphoma-associated HLH, and 12% for those with NK/T-cell lymphoma-associated HLH.[39] Increasing age had an independent negative impact on survival within EBV-associated or B-cell lymphoma-associated HLH. Consistent findings were increased early mortality in patients with underlying malignancy (eg, median OS 1.1 vs 47 months and 1.4 vs 23 months), increased age, and decreased platelet count less than 40×10^9/L.[56] Occasionally cited adverse factors were male sex, splenomegaly, active EBV infection, fever not subsiding within 3 days of diagnosis, disseminated intravascular coagulation, hypoalbuminemia, and lack of etoposide during management.[57] Ferritin levels greater than 50,000 ng/mL have been a predictor for 30-day mortality (hazard ratio, 3.3).[42]

Systematic analyses of efficacy for therapies in adults with HLH are lacking. A review of nine therapeutic studies revealed wide variation in practice; most trials used steroids and intravenous immunoglobulin with few patients undergoing the HLH-94 protocol.[47] In a Japanese study of more than 200 adults, those with EBV-associated HLH were treated with therapies ranging from steroids or intravenous immunoglobulin alone, to the HLH-94 regimen, to multidrug chemotherapy.[39] Only six patients received stem cell transplantation for infection-associated HLH. In this study, 132 adults had malignancy-associated HLH. Patients with lymphoma-associated HLH received multidrug chemotherapy with CHOP ± etoposide ± rituximab. Six of 32 patients with NK/T-cell lymphoma underwent HSCT (two autologous, four allogeneic) with 3-year OS of 50% versus 10% without HSCT. Ten of 47 patients with B-cell lymphoma underwent HSCT (eight autologous, two allogeneic), with 3-year OS of 79% versus 48% without HSCT. Samples sizes were too small to show a significant survival difference. A French study of 162 adults with HLH revealed that 38% of patients did not receive any specific treatment of HLH and instead were treated for the underlying disease. Immunosuppressive therapy consisted primarily of steroids, with etoposide administered in first- or second-line in 50% of patients.[56] There was a trend to improved survival in patients who received etoposide (85% vs 74%; $P = .08$), respectively. There was no comment on use of HSCT. Other large retrospective analyses of adults with HLH confirm the variation in underlying etiologies and therapies used. Few adults underwent HSCT.[42,44,58,59]

Most information on using HSCT in adult-onset HLH is in the form of case reports and very preliminary data from the Center for International Blood and Marrow Transplant Research. Older reports indicate success after autologous stem cell transplantation in B-cell, T-cell, and NK/T-cell lymphoma-associated HLH.[60–63] Successful examples of allogeneic HSCT include a young woman with anaplastic large-cell lymphoma and HLH treated with modified HLH-94 protocol and allogeneic HSCT, a patient with NK/T-cell lymphoma and HLH treated with allogeneic MUD HSCT, and a 62 year old with angioimmunoblastic T-cell lymphoma with HLH who underwent RIC MUD HSCT.[64–66] Given the dearth of information, we queried the Center for International Blood and Marrow Transplant Research as to outcomes of adults receiving allogeneic transplants for histiocytic diseases.[67] Preliminary data indicate 47 adult patients underwent allogeneic HSCT between 2001 and 2012. Median age was 25 years (range, 18–67); 37 were categorized as having familial or acquired HLH. Donors included 15 MRDs, 1 haploidentical, 30 MUDs, and 1 UCB unit. Twenty-six (56%) received myeloablative and 21 (44%) received RIC. Alemtuzumab was included in conditioning of 18 subjects (38%). Survival estimates for the entire cohort were 93% at 100 days, 60% at 1 year, and 57% at 2 years after HSCT. Although additional details are needed, it seems that allogeneic HSCT is feasible and worthy of further systematic investigation in adults with HLH.

LACK OF A CLEAR ALGORITHM IN ADULT-ONSET HEMOPHAGOCYTIC LYMPHOHISTIOCYTOSIS

Given the myriad underlying causes for adult-onset HLH including inherited hypomorphic or heterozygous mutations and variants, malignancy, infection, and rheumatologic disease, initial approaches have focused on treating the underlying conditions. Standardized approaches have not been studied, and data on who will benefit from HSCT as consolidation are not available. Extrapolating from the pediatric literature and anecdotal experiences at our institution, one potential adult algorithm is proposed next and in **Fig. 2**.

1. For a patient with a history of recurrent infections and inflammatory complications and variants in classical familial HLH genes, we follow the HLH-2004 protocol and consolidate with allogeneic HSCT. An example is a 35-year-old woman with a history of severe infections since childhood and autoimmune lymphoproliferative syndrome and who is heterozygous for two variants in syntaxin binding protein 2

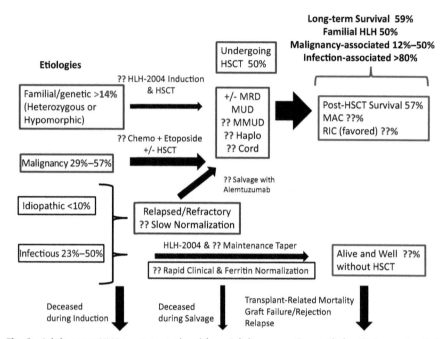

Fig. 2. Adult-onset HLH treatment algorithm. Adults presenting with familial or potentially genetically driven HLH are considered for HSCT after induction therapy. How to manage those who have atypical variants or are only heterozygous for "causative" mutations in HLH-associated genes is unknown. Adults with malignancy underlying HLH are generally considered for multiagent chemotherapy containing etoposide. Often upfront allogeneic HSCT is considered if not already indicated for the malignancy itself. The role of alemtuzumab in salvage and periconditioning therapy for adults is unproven. Whether rate of normalization of clinical and laboratory abnormalities, specifically ferritin, in patients with idiopathic or infection-associated HLH should impact decisions to proceed with HSCT or maintenance of immune suppression is unclear. If HSCT is needed, current preferences are to use reduced-intensity conditioning and a fully matched unrelated donor. Use of an asymptomatic matched sibling adult donor who carries a potentially predisposing variant can be considered if a matched unrelated donor is not available. More data on conditioning intensities and alternative donor choices are needed. ??, indicates areas where more data are needed to inform clinical decision-making; Cord, umbilical cord unit; Haplo, haploidentical donor.

(STXBP2). One mutation is known to be causative in the homozygous state and the other is a previously undocumented deletion resulting in a premature stop codon. She was treated with HLH-2004, relapsed during maintenance therapy, was salvaged with alemtuzumab, and underwent RIC MUD HSCT.

2. For a patient with lymphoma underlying HLH, etoposide is preferred in a multiagent chemotherapy regimen. Serious consideration is given to consolidative allogeneic HSCT particularly in the case of T-cell or NK/T-cell lymphomas if a matched donor can be identified. An example is a 38-year-old man with gamma-delta panniculitis-like T-cell lymphoma, which is known to have a poor prognosis in concert with HLH. He received etoposide-containing chemotherapy with resolution of his symptoms and PET scan and then underwent RIC MRD HSCT. He was incidentally found to be heterozygous for a variant in STXBP2 found at a frequency of 0.4% in the healthy population.

3. For a patient with no underlying genetic abnormality detected and no underlying malignancy, HLH-2004 therapy is pursued. In patients whose clinical symptoms and ferritin quickly normalize and remain normal as maintenance therapy is tapered off, calcineurin inhibition is continued for at least a year. Those who do not tolerate taper of etoposide and steroids receive RIC HSCT. An example is a 65-year-old man with HLH whose infectious, malignant, and genetic work-up was negative and who had resolution of clinical and laboratory parameters within 2 weeks of starting HLH-2004 therapy. He is now maintained on a calcineurin inhibitor with normal ferritin.

Additional complexities are often introduced rather than clarified by advanced genetic testing. The approach to adults who present with idiopathic HLH, normalize quickly with therapy, but harbor variations in familial HLH genes of unclear prognostic import, such as PRF1 A91V, is undetermined. Adult patients who are heterozygous for genetic variants and mutations are likely to have sibling donors harboring the same variants. Whether to preferentially select an asymptomatic adult MRD with a potentially predisposing variant or MUD is unknown. Adults tend to have higher TRM than children, particularly with use of alternative donors, so the role for haploidentical donors and umbilical cord stem cells in this setting is unclear.

SUMMARY

The role of reduced-intensity allogeneic HSCT from a variety of donor sources in improving survival for children with familial HLH is well-documented. The minority of children with infection-associated HLH need HSCT, but salvage therapy with alemtuzumab and consolidative allogeneic HSCT for those with refractory or relapsed disease is clearly indicated. Optimal peritransplant dosing of alemtuzumab for improved donor chimerism and clinical outcomes is under investigation. The heterogeneity of adult-onset HLH has complicated evaluation of initial therapy and of HSCT as definitive treatment. Therapy for adults with HLH is often individualized, but institutions are now generating algorithms that include HSCT based on growing experience. Consolidation of these data is desperately needed to optimize management of the growing number of adults recognized to have HLH and to achieve dramatic improvements in survival like those attained in pediatric HLH over the past two decades.

REFERENCES

1. Farquhar J, Claireaux A. Familial haemophagocytic reticulosis. Arch Dis Child 1952;27(136):519–25.
2. Filipovich AH. The expanding spectrum of hemophagocytic lymphohistiocytosis. Curr Opin Allergy Clin Immunol 2011;11(6):512–6.
3. Henter J-I, Samuelsson-Horne A, Aricò M, et al. Treatment of hemophagocytic lymphohistiocytosis with HLH-94 immunochemotherapy and bone marrow transplantation. Blood 2002;100(7):2367–73.
4. Trottestam H, Horne A, Aricò M, et al. Chemoimmunotherapy for hemophagocytic lymphohistiocytosis: long-term results of the HLH-94 treatment protocol. Blood 2011;118(17):4577–84.
5. Lin TF, Ferlic-Stark LL, Allen CE, et al. Rate of decline of ferritin in patients with hemophagocytic lymphohistiocytosis as a prognostic variable for mortality. Pediatr Blood Cancer 2011;56(1):154–5.

6. Henter J-I, Horne A, Aricó M, et al. HLH-2004: diagnostic and therapeutic guidelines for hemophagocytic lymphohistiocytosis. Pediatr Blood Cancer 2007;48(2): 124–31.

7. Stephan J, Donadieu J, Ledeist F, et al. Treatment of familial hemophagocytic lymphohistiocytosis with antithymocyte globulins, steroids, and cyclosporin A. Blood 1993;82(8):2319–23.

8. Mahlaoui N, Ouachée-Chardin M, de Saint Basile G, et al. Immunotherapy of familial hemophagocytic lymphohistiocytosis with antithymocyte globulins: a single-center retrospective report of 38 patients. Pediatrics 2007;120(3):e622–8.

9. Gilleece MH, Dexter TM. Effect of Campath-1H antibody on human hematopoietic progenitors in vitro. Blood 1993;82(3):807–12.

10. Strout MP, Seropian S, Berliner N. Alemtuzumab as a bridge to allogeneic SCT in atypical hemophagocytic lymphohistiocytosis. Nat Rev Clin Oncol 2010;7(7): 415–20.

11. Marsh RA, Allen CE, McClain KL, et al. Salvage therapy of refractory hemophagocytic lymphohistiocytosis with alemtuzumab. Pediatr Blood Cancer 2013; 60(1):101–9.

12. Henzan T, Nagafuji K, Tsukamoto H, et al. Success with infliximab in treating refractory hemophagocytic lymphohistiocytosis. Am J Hematol 2006;81(1):59–61.

13. Rajasekaran S, Kruse K, Kovey K, et al. Therapeutic role of anakinra, an interleukin-1 receptor antagonist, in the management of secondary hemophagocytic lymphohistiocytosis/sepsis/multiple organ dysfunction/macrophage activating syndrome in critically Ill children. Pediatr Crit Care Med 2014;15(5):401–8.

14. Kelly A, Ramanan AV. A case of macrophage activation syndrome successfully treated with anakinra. Nat Clin Pract Rheumatol 2008;4(11):615–20.

15. Olin RL, Nichols KE, Naghashpour M, et al. Successful use of the anti-CD25 antibody daclizumab in an adult patient with hemophagocytic lymphohistiocytosis. Am J Hematol 2008;83(9):747–9.

16. Zhang L-J, Zhang S-J, Xu J, et al. Splenectomy for an adult patient with refractory secondary hemophagocytic lymphohistiocytosis. Biomed Pharmacother 2011; 65(6):432–5.

17. Fischer A, Cerf-Bensussan N, Blanche S, et al. Allogeneic bone marrow transplantation for erythrophagocytic lymphohistiocytosis. J Pediatr 1986;108(2):267–70.

18. Blanche S, Caniglia M, Girault D, et al. Treatment of hemophagocytic lymphohistiocytosis with chemotherapy and bone marrow transplantation: a single-center study of 22 cases. Blood 1991;78(1):51–4.

19. Ouachée-Chardin M, Elie C, de Saint Basile G, et al. Hematopoietic stem cell transplantation in hemophagocytic lymphohistiocytosis: a single-center report of 48 patients. Pediatrics 2006;117(4):e743–50.

20. Hale GA, Bowman LC, Woodard JP, et al. Allogeneic bone marrow transplantation for children with histiocytic disorders: use of TBI and omission of etoposide in the conditioning regimen. Bone Marrow Transplant 2003;31(11):981–6.

21. Naithani R, Asim M, Naqvi A, et al. Increased complications and morbidity in children with hemophagocytic lymphohistiocytosis undergoing hematopoietic stem cell transplantation. Clin Transplant 2013;27(2):248–54.

22. Baker KS, DeLaat CA, Steinbuch M, et al. Successful correction of hemophagocytic lymphohistiocytosis with related or unrelated bone marrow transplantation. Blood 1997;89(10):3857–63.

23. Horne A, Janka G, Maarten Egeler R, et al. Haematopoietic stem cell transplantation in haemophagocytic lymphohistiocytosis. Br J Haematol 2005;129(5): 622–30.

24. Baker KS, Filipovich AH, Gross TG, et al. Unrelated donor hematopoietic cell transplantation for hemophagocytic lymphohistiocytosis. Bone Marrow Transplant 2008;42(3):175–80.
25. Cooper N, Rao K, Gilmour K, et al. Stem cell transplantation with reduced-intensity conditioning for hemophagocytic lymphohistiocytosis. Blood 2006; 107(3):1233–6.
26. Cooper N, Rao K, Goulden N, et al. The use of reduced-intensity stem cell transplantation in haemophagocytic lymphohistiocytosis and Langerhans cell histiocytosis. Bone Marrow Transplant 2008;42(Suppl 2):S47–50.
27. Marsh RA, Jordan MB, Filipovich AH. Reduced-intensity conditioning haematopoietic cell transplantation for haemophagocytic lymphohistiocytosis: an important step forward. Br J Haematol 2011;154(5):556–63.
28. Ohga S, Kudo K, Ishii E, et al. Hematopoietic stem cell transplantation for familial hemophagocytic lymphohistiocytosis and Epstein–Barr virus-associated hemophagocytic lymphohistiocytosis in Japan. Pediatr Blood Cancer 2010;54(2): 299–306.
29. Hamidieh AA, Pourpak Z, Yari K, et al. Hematopoietic stem cell transplantation with a reduced-intensity conditioning regimen in pediatric patients with Griscelli syndrome type 2. Pediatr Transplant 2013;17(5):487–91.
30. Lehmberg K, Albert MH, Beier R, et al. Treosulfan-based conditioning regimen for children and adolescents with hemophagocytic lymphohistiocytosis. Blood 2014; 99(1):180–4.
31. Yoon HS, Im HJ, Moon HN, et al. The outcome of hematopoietic stem cell transplantation in Korean children with hemophagocytic lymphohistiocytosis. Pediatr Transplant 2010;14(6):735–40.
32. Nishi M, Nishimura R, Suzuki N, et al. Reduced-intensity conditioning in unrelated donor cord blood transplantation for familial hemophagocytic lymphohistiocytosis. Am J Hematol 2012;87(6):637–9.
33. Marsh RA, Vaughn G, Kim M-O, et al. Reduced-intensity conditioning significantly improves survival of patients with hemophagocytic lymphohistiocytosis undergoing allogeneic hematopoietic cell transplantation. Blood 2010;116(26): 5824–31.
34. Marsh RA, Kim M-O, Liu C, et al. An intermediate alemtuzumab schedule reduces the incidence of mixed chimerism following reduced-intensity conditioning hematopoietic cell transplantation for hemophagocytic lymphohistiocytosis. Biol Blood Marrow Transplant 2013;19(11):1625–31.
35. Booth C, Gilmour KC, Veys P, et al. X-linked lymphoproliferative disease due to SAP/SH2D1A deficiency: a multicenter study on the manifestations, management and outcome of the disease. Blood 2011;117(1):53–62.
36. Marsh RA, Bleesing JJ, Chandrakasan S, et al. Reduced-intensity conditioning hematopoietic cell transplantation is an effective treatment for patients with SLAM-associated protein deficiency/X-linked lymphoproliferative disease type 1. Biol Blood Marrow Transplant 2014;20(10):1641–5.
37. Marsh RA, Rao K, Satwani P, et al. Allogeneic hematopoietic cell transplantation for XIAP deficiency: an international survey reveals poor outcomes. Blood 2013; 121(6):877–83.
38. Imashuku S, Teramura T, Tauchi H, et al. Longitudinal follow-up of patients with Epstein-Barr virus-associated hemophagocytic lymphohistiocytosis. Haematologica 2004;89(2):183–8.
39. Ishii E, Ohga S, Imashuku S, et al. Nationwide survey of hemophagocytic lymphohistiocytosis in Japan. Int J Hematol 2007;86(1):58–65.

40. Giri P, Pal P, Ghosh A, et al. Infection-associated haemophagocytic lymphohistio-cytosis: a case series using steroids only protocol for management. Rheumatol Int 2013;33(5):1363–6.
41. Imashuku S, Kuriyama K, Teramura T, et al. Requirement for etoposide in the treatment of Epstein-Barr virus–associated hemophagocytic lymphohistiocytosis. J Clin Oncol 2001;19(10):2665–73.
42. Parikh SA, Kapoor P, Letendre L, et al. Prognostic factors and outcomes of adults with hemophagocytic lymphohistiocytosis. Mayo Clinic Proc 2014;89(4):484–92.
43. Li J, Wang Q, Zheng W, et al. Hemophagocytic lymphohistiocytosis: clinical anal-ysis of 103 adult patients. Medicine 2014;93(2):100–5.
44. Otrock ZK, Eby CS. Clinical characteristics, prognostic factors, and outcomes of adult patients with hemophagocytic lymphohistiocytosis. Am J Hematol 2015; 90(3):220–4.
45. Fardet L, Galicier L, Lambotte O, et al. Development and validation of the HScore, a score for the diagnosis of reactive hemophagocytic syndrome. Arthritis Rheu-matol 2014;66(9):2613–20.
46. Tang Y, Xu X, Song H, et al. Early diagnostic and prognostic significance of a spe-cific Th1/Th2 cytokine pattern in children with haemophagocytic syndrome. Br J Haematol 2008;143(1):84–91.
47. Ramos-Casals M, Brito-Zerón P, López-Guillermo A, et al. Adult haemophago-cytic syndrome. Lancet 2014;383(9927):1503–16.
48. Machaczka M, Vaktnäs J, Klimkowska M, et al. Malignancy-associated hemopha-gocytic lymphohistiocytosis in adults: a retrospective population-based analysis from a single center. Leuk Lymphoma 2011;52(4):613–9.
49. Wang Y, Wang Z, Zhang J, et al. Genetic features of late onset primary hemopha-gocytic lymphohistiocytosis in adolescence or adulthood. PLoS One 2014;9(9): e107386.
50. Ueda I, Ishii E, Morimoto A, et al. Correlation between phenotypic heterogeneity and gene mutational characteristics in familial hemophagocytic lymphohistiocy-tosis (FHL). Pediatr Blood Cancer 2006;46(4):482–8.
51. Pagel J, Beutel K, Lehmberg K, et al. Distinct mutations in STXBP2 are associ-ated with variable clinical presentations in patients with familial hemophagocytic lymphohistiocytosis type 5 (FHL5). Blood 2012;119(25):6016–24.
52. Zhang K, Jordan MB, Marsh RA, et al. Hypomorphic mutations in PRF1, MUNC13-4, and STXBP2 are associated with adult-onset familial HLH. Blood 2011;118(22):5794–8.
53. Manso R, Rodríguez-Pinilla SM, Lombardia L, et al. An A91V SNP in the *Perforin* Gene Is Frequently Found in NK/T-Cell Lymphomas. PLoS ONE 2014;9(3):e91521.
54. House IG, Thia K, Brennan AJ, et al. Heterozygosity for the common perforin mu-tation, p.A91V, impairs the cytotoxicity of primary natural killer cells from healthy individuals. Immunol Cell Biol 2015;93(6):575–80.
55. Martínez-Pomar N, Lanio N, Romo N, et al. Functional impact of A91V mutation of the PRF1 perforin gene. Hum Immunol 2013;74(1):14–7.
56. Arca M, Fardet L, Galicier L, et al. Prognostic factors of early death in a cohort of 162 adult haemophagocytic syndrome: impact of triggering disease and early treatment with etoposide. Br J Haematol 2015;168(1):63–8.
57. Tseng Y-T, Sheng W-H, Lin B-H, et al. Causes, clinical symptoms, and outcomes of infectious diseases associated with hemophagocytic lymphohistiocytosis in Taiwanese adults. J Microbiol Immunol Infect 2011;44(3):191–7.
58. Park H-S, Kim D-Y, Lee J-H, et al. Clinical features of adult patients with second-ary hemophagocytic lymphohistiocytosis from causes other than lymphoma: an

analysis of treatment outcome and prognostic factors. Ann Hematol 2012;91(6): 897–904.

59. Rivière S, Galicier L, Coppo P, et al. Reactive hemophagocytic syndrome in adults: a retrospective analysis of 162 patients. Am J Med 2014;127(11):1118–25.

60. Takami A, Nakao S, Ueda M, et al. Successful treatment of B-cell lymphoma associated with hemophagocytic syndrome using autologous peripheral blood CD34 positive cell transplantation followed by induction of autologous graft-versus-host disease. Ann Hematol 2000;79(7):389–91.

61. Hirai H, Shimazaki C, Hatsuse M, et al. Autologous peripheral blood stem cell transplantation for adult patients with B-cell lymphoma-associated hemophagocytic syndrome. Leukemia 2001;15(2):311.

62. Jassal DS, Kasper K, Morales C, et al. Autologous peripheral stem cell transplantation for aggressive hemophagocytic syndrome associated with T-cell lymphoma: case study and review. Am J Hematol 2002;69(1):64–6.

63. Inoue D, Nagai Y, Takiuchi Y, et al. Successful treatment of extranodal natural killer/T-cell lymphoma, nasal type, complicated by severe hemophagocytic syndrome, with dexamethasone, methotrexate, ifosfamide, l-asparaginase, and etoposide chemotherapy followed by autologous stem cell transplant. Leuk Lymphoma 2010;51(4):720–3.

64. Machaczka M, Nahi H, Karbach H, et al. Successful treatment of recurrent malignancy-associated hemophagocytic lymphohistiocytosis with a modified HLH-94 immunochemotherapy and allogeneic stem cell transplantation. Med Oncol 2012;29(2):1231–6.

65. Yun S, Taverna JA, Puvvada SD, et al. NK/T-cell non-Hodgkin's lymphoma with secondary haemophagocytic lymphohistiocytosis treated with matched unrelated donor allogeneic stem cell transplant. BMJ Case Rep 2014;2014. [Epub ahead of print].

66. Yu J-T, Hwang W-L, Wang R-C, et al. Reduced intensity conditioning allogeneic hematopoietic stem cell transplant could be beneficial to angioimmunoblastic T-cell lymphoma patients with hemophagocytic lymphohistiocytosis. Ann Hematol 2012;91(5):805–7.

67. Nikiforow S, Korman S, Eapen M, et al. Outcomes after allogeneic stem cell transplantation in adults for histiocytic disorders including hemophagocytic lymphohistiocytosis. Biol Blood Marrow Transplant 2014;20(2 Suppl 1):S243. abstracts from 2014 BMT tandem meetings.

Index

Note: Page numbers of article titles are in **boldface** type.

Hematol Oncol Clin N Am 29 (2015) 961–970
http://dx.doi.org/10.1016/S0889-8588(15)00130-6
0889-8588/15/$ – see front matter © 2015 Elsevier Inc. All rights reserved.

United States Postal Service

Statement of Ownership, Management, and Circulation
(All Periodicals Publications Except Requester Publications)

1. Publication Title	2. Publication Number	3. Filing Date
Hematology/Oncology Clinics of North America	0 0 0 2 - 4 7 3 3	9/18/15

4. Issue Frequency	5. Number of Issues Published Annually	6. Annual Subscription Price
Feb, Apr, Jun, Aug, Oct, Dec	6	$385.00

7. Complete Mailing Address of Known Office of Publication (Not printer) (Street, city, county, state, and ZIP+48®)

Elsevier Inc.
360 Park Avenue South
New York, NY 10010-1710

Contact Person
Stephen R. Bushing
Telephone (Include area code)
215-239-3688

8. Complete Mailing Address of Headquarters or General Business Office of Publisher (Not printer)

Elsevier Inc., 360 Park Avenue South, New York, NY 10010-1710

9. Full Names and Complete Mailing Addresses of Publisher, Editor, and Managing Editor (Do not leave blank)

Publisher (Name and complete mailing address)

Linda Belfus, Elsevier Inc., 1600 John F. Kennedy Blvd., Suite 1800, Philadelphia, PA 19103

Editor (Name and complete mailing address)

Jennifer Flynn-Briggs, Elsevier Inc., 1600 John F. Kennedy Blvd., Suite 1800, Philadelphia, PA 19103-2899

Managing Editor (Name and complete mailing address)

Adrianne Brigido, Elsevier Inc., 1600 John F. Kennedy Blvd., Suite 1800, Philadelphia, PA 19103-2899

10. Owner (Do not leave blank. If the publication is owned by a corporation, give the name and address of the corporation immediately followed by the names and addresses of all stockholders owning or holding 1 percent or more of the total amount of stock. If not owned by a corporation, give the names and addresses of the individual owners. If owned by a partnership or other unincorporated firm, give its name and address as well as those of each individual owner. If the publication is published by a nonprofit organization, give its name and address.)

Full Name	Complete Mailing Address
Wholly owned subsidiary of	1600 John F. Kennedy Blvd, Ste. 1800
Reed/Elsevier, US holdings	Philadelphia, PA 19103-2899

11. Known Bondholders, Mortgagees, and Other Security Holders Owning or Holding 1 Percent or More of Total Amount of Bonds, Mortgages, or Other Securities. If none, check box ☐ None

Full Name	Complete Mailing Address
N/A	

12. Tax Status (For completion by nonprofit organizations authorized to mail at nonprofit rates) (Check one)
The purpose, function, and nonprofit status of this organization and the exempt status for federal income tax purposes:
☐ Has Not Changed During Preceding 12 Months
☐ Has Changed During Preceding 12 Months (Publisher must submit explanation of change with this statement)

13. Publication Title	14. Issue Date for Circulation Data Below
Hematology/Oncology Clinics of North America	August 2015

PS Form 3526, July 2014 (Page 1 of 3 (Instructions Page 3)) PSN 7530-01-000-9931 PRIVACY NOTICE: See our Privacy policy in www.usps.com

15.	Extent and Nature of Circulation		Average No. Copies Each Issue During Preceding 12 Months	No. Copies of Single Issue Published Nearest to Filing Date
a. Total Number of Copies (Net press run)			638	542
b. Legitimate Paid and/Or Requested Distribution (By Mail and Outside the Mail)	(1)	Mailed Outside County Paid/Requested Mail Subscriptions stated on PS Form 3541. (Include paid distribution above nominal rate, advertiser's proof copies and exchange copies)	185	155
	(2)	Mailed In-County Paid/Requested Mail Subscriptions stated on PS Form 3541. (Include paid distribution above nominal rate, advertiser's proof copies and exchange copies)	111	143
	(3)	Paid Distribution Outside the Mails Including Sales Through Dealers And Carriers, Street Vendors, Counter Sales, and Other Paid Distribution Outside USPS®		
	(4)	Paid Distribution by Other Classes of Mail Through the USPS (e.g. First-Class Mail®)		
c. Total Paid and or Requested Distribution (Sum of 15b (1), (2), (3), and (4))		▲	296	298
d. Free or Nominal Rate Distribution (By Mail and Outside the Mail)	(1)	Free or Nominal Rate Outside-County Copies included on PS Form 3541	131	127
	(2)	Free or Nominal Rate In-County Copies included on PS Form 3541		
	(3)	Free or Nominal Rate Copies mailed at Other classes Through the USPS (e.g. First-Class Mail®)		
	(4)	Free or Nominal Rate Distribution Outside the Mail (Carriers or Other means)		
e. Total Nonrequested Distribution (Sum of 15d (1), (2), (3) and (4))		▲	131	127
f. Total Distribution (Sum of 15c and 15e)		▲	427	425
g. Copies not Distributed (See instructions to publishers #4 (page #3))		▲	211	117
h. Total (Sum of 15f and g)			638	542
i. Percent Paid and/or Requested Circulation (15c divided by 15f times 100)		▲	69.32%	70.12%

16. Electronic Copy Circulation	Average No. Copies Each Issue During Preceding 12 Months	No. Copies of Single Issue Published Nearest to Filing Date
a. Paid Electronic Copies		
b. Total paid Print Copies (Line 15c) + Paid Electronic copies (Line 16a)		
c. Total Print Distribution (Line 15f) + Paid Electronic Copies (Line 16a)		
d. Percent Paid (Both Print & Electronic copies) (16b divided by 16c X 100)		

☐ I certify that 50% of all my distributed copies (electronic and print) are paid above a nominal price.

17. Publication of Statement of Ownership
If the publication is a general publication, publication of this statement is required. Will be printed in the October 2015 issue of this publication.

18. Signature and Title of Editor, Publisher, Business Manager, or Owner

Date: September 18, 2015

Stephen R. Bushing
Stephen R. Bushing – Inventory Distribution Coordinator

I certify that all information furnished on this form is true and complete. I understand that anyone who furnishes false or misleading information on this form or who omits material or information requested on the form may be subject to criminal sanctions (including fines and imprisonment) and/or civil sanctions (including civil penalties).

PS Form 3526, July 2014 (Page 3 of 3)

Moving?

Make sure your subscription moves with you!

To notify us of your new address, find your **Clinics Account Number** (located on your mailing label above your name), and contact customer service at:

Email: journalscustomerservice-usa@elsevier.com

800-654-2452 (subscribers in the U.S. & Canada)
314-447-8871 (subscribers outside of the U.S. & Canada)

Fax number: 314-447-8029

Elsevier Health Sciences Division
Subscription Customer Service
3251 Riverport Lane
Maryland Heights, MO 63043

*To ensure uninterrupted delivery of your subscription, please notify us at least 4 weeks in advance of move.

Printed and bound by CPI Group (UK) Ltd, Croydon, CR0 4YY

03/10/2024

01040485-0015